SHAOLIN INVINCIBLE

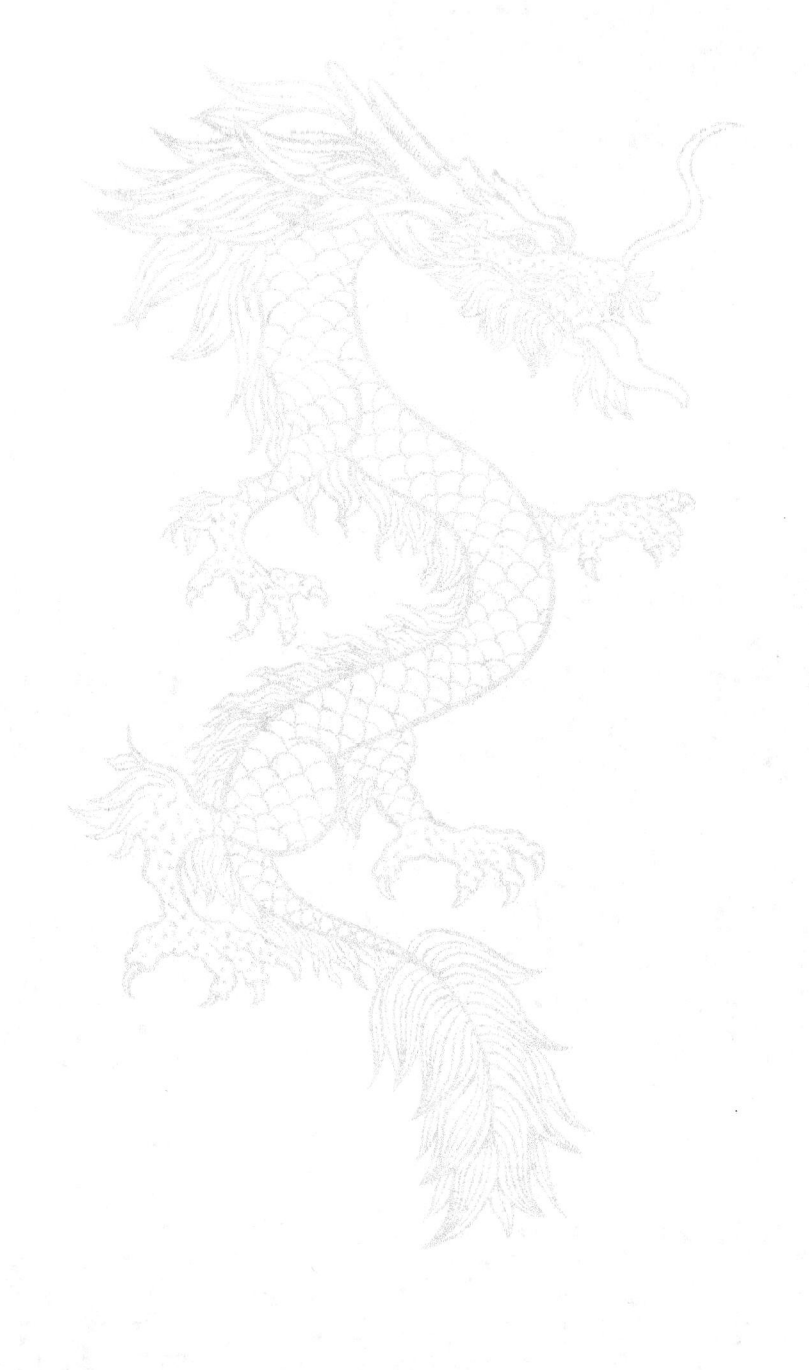

SHAOLIN INVINCIBLE

The martial arts manifesto on finding the warrior within you

Denis Ark

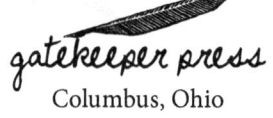

Columbus, Ohio

Shaolin Invincible: The martial arts manifesto on finding the warrior within you

Published by Gatekeeper Press
2167 Stringtown Rd., Suite 109
Columbus, OH 43123-2989
www.GatekeeperPress.com

Copyright © 2022 by Denis Ark
All rights reserved. Neither this book, nor any parts within it may be sold or reproduced in any form or by any electronic or mechanical means, including information storage and retrieval systems without permission in writing from the author. The only exception is by a reviewer, who may quote short excerpts in a review.

The cover design, interior formatting, typesetting, and editorial work for this book are entirely the product of the author. Gatekeeper Press did not participate in and is not responsible for any aspect of these elements.

Copyright for the images: iStockphoto.com/NikolaVukojevic (torn paper), ilonitta (Chinese dragon pattern)
Library of Congress Control Number: 2021948757
ISBN (paperback): 9781662918995
eISBN: 9781662913426

CONTENTS

DISCLAIMER IX

REFERENCE ACKNOWLEDGEMENT XI

PREFACE XIII

    EVERYTHING ZEN XV

    THE ULTIMATE WARRIOR XXI

    THE LITTLE DRAGON TAKES FLIGHT XXVII

INTRODUCTION XXXIII

    THE POWER WITHIN YOU XXXV

    POWER-CONSCIOUSNESS XLI

    THE MOTIVE DRIVES POWER XLV

    THE NINE GATES TO INVINCIBILITY XLVII

THE GRASSHOPPER XLIX

GATE 1—MARTIAL ARTS LI

    CHAPTER 1: WHAT ARE MARTIAL ARTS? 1

    CHAPTER 2: NATURE AWAITS YOUR DIRECTION 9

    CHAPTER 3: WHO IS YOUR MASTER? 15

    CHAPTER 4: EVERYONE WANTS TO BE BRUCE LEE 25

    CHAPTER 5: THE WARRIOR SPIRIT 39

    GATE 1 KEY POINTS 49

THE TIGER	**51**
GATE 2—THE FOUR FACTORS OF FITNESS	**53**
CHAPTER 6: STRENGTH	63
CHAPTER 7: FLEXIBILITY	71
CHAPTER 8: CONDITIONING	77
CHAPTER 9: NUTRITION	99
GATE 2—KEY POINTS	115
THE DRAGON	**117**
GATE 3—INTERNAL ENERGY	**119**
CHAPTER 10: POWER IN PROVIDENCE	125
CHAPTER 11: POWER IN ALLIANCE	131
CHAPTER 12: POWER IN PRACTICE	137
CHAPTER 13: PHYSICAL POWER	143
CHAPTER 14: MENTAL POWER	163
CHAPTER 15: SPIRITUAL POWER	173
GATE 3 KEY POINTS	179
EPILOGUE	**181**
ABOUT THE AUTHOR	**183**
ENDNOTES	**185**
REFERENCES	**195**

I offer my deepest gratitude to the masters and teachers who passed down their knowledge, infusing my life with their wisdom.

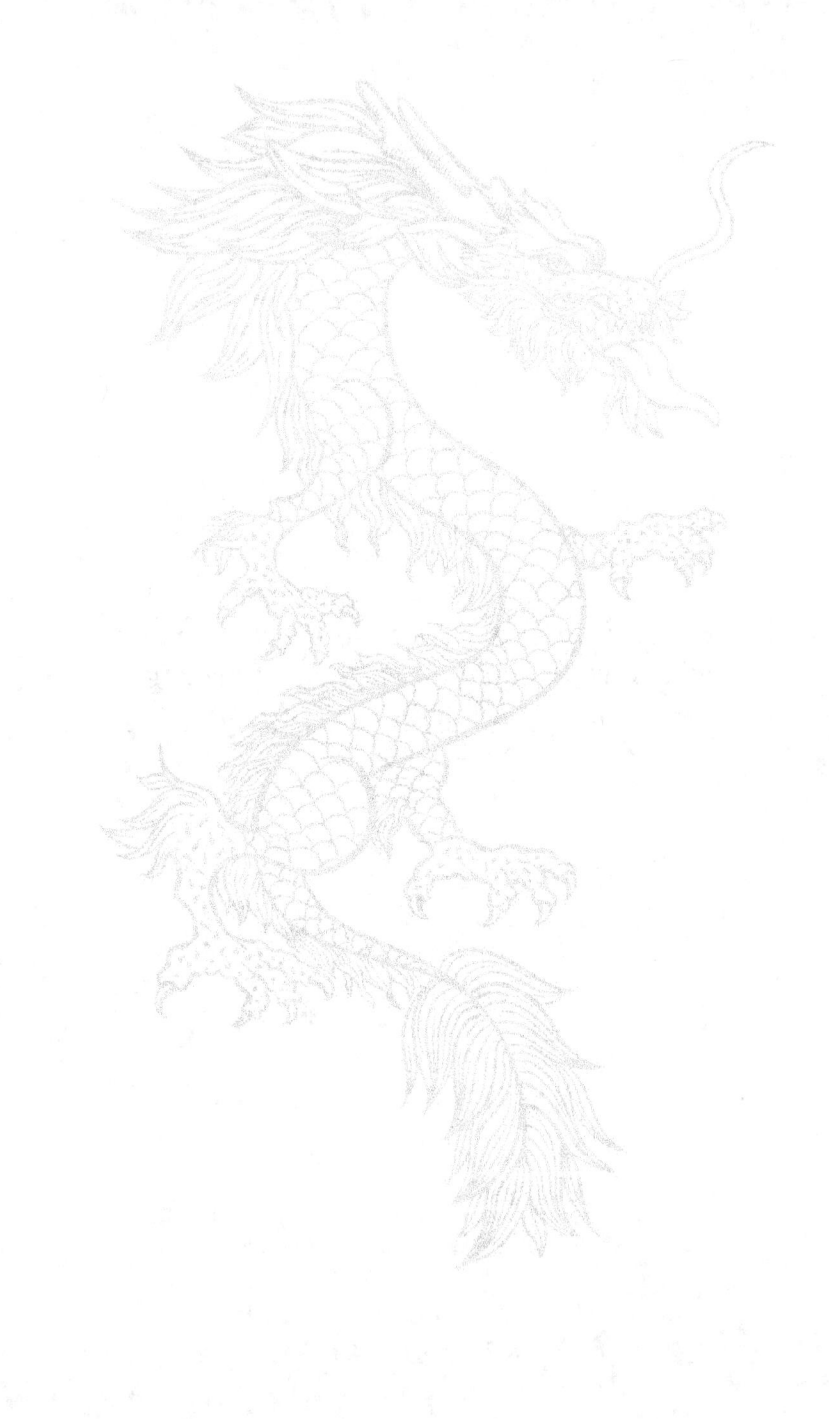

DISCLAIMER

Please read this book at your discretion. Although anyone may find the methods, practices, and philosophies in this book useful, all of the content within is available under the understanding that neither the author nor the publisher is engaged in presenting specific emotional, psychological, physical, medical, sexual, or spiritual advice. Nothing in this book constitutes a recommendation, prescription, diagnosis, or cure for any emotional, psychological, physical, nutritional, medical, sexual, or spiritual problem.

The author of this material is not responsible in any manner whatsoever for any injury, illness, or death that may occur through reading or following the instructions in this manual. The activities (physical, mental, spiritual, or otherwise) described in this material may be too strenuous or dangerous for some people. The reader should consult with a physician before engaging in them.

Every individual has specific needs, and this book cannot take these individual differences into account. Any reader who needs particular help should engage in a program of prevention, treatment, cure, or general health and nutrition—only in consultation with a licensed, qualified nutritionist, physician, therapist, or other certified professional. Any person suffering from a psychological condition, disease, or illness should consult a medical practitioner.

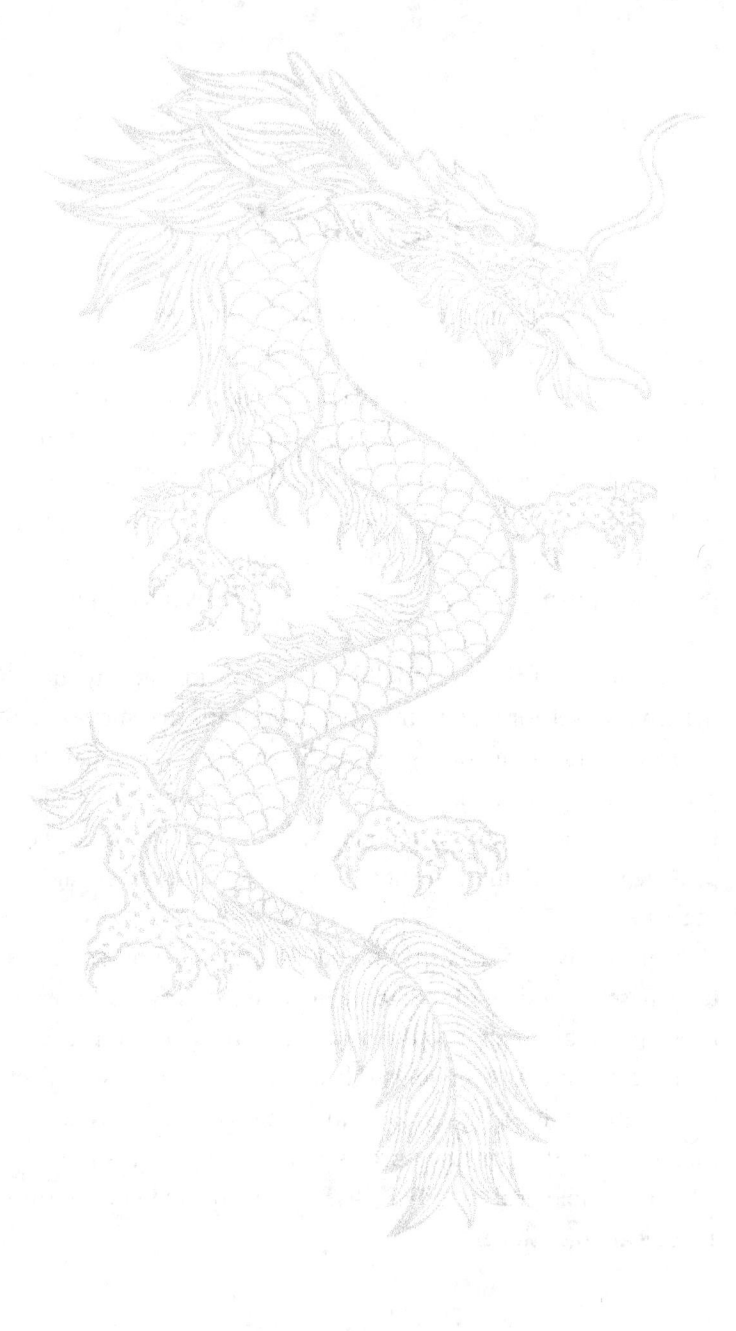

REFERENCE ACKNOWLEDGEMENT

This manuscript as a whole is a personal manifesto of my life experiences through twenty-five years of research and practice. The information comes from many different sources across various fields including martial arts, bodybuilding, nutrition, science, religion, and philosophy, all of which are now wrapped up into a big ball within me.

Many of the ideas contained within this book were passed on to me from my teachers, as well as learned during my time in Hong Kong where I studied Eastern techniques and philosophies. A plethora of martial-arts information comes from my martial-arts lineage, and is well-known throughout the various kung fu schools in the world.

In addition, I used to frequent the Chaung Yen Monastery in Upstate New York, where during weekly lectures I learned about Zen Buddhism and how to meditate and heal the mind and body.

In this book, I frequently talk about "the natural laws," most of which are hermetic laws and religious concepts well-known around the world. These can be independently researched. However, they are also mixed in with my own interpretations and conclusions. Where this is the case, I will inform the reader.

As this is my life's work, it is difficult to formally reference each source, but I would like to thank every teacher and source who has contributed to this book. If you would like to be formally referenced for an idea, please notify me via email and I will update this in a subsequent edition.

May this book serve you on your path, and may you become your best version to benefit others.

PREFACE

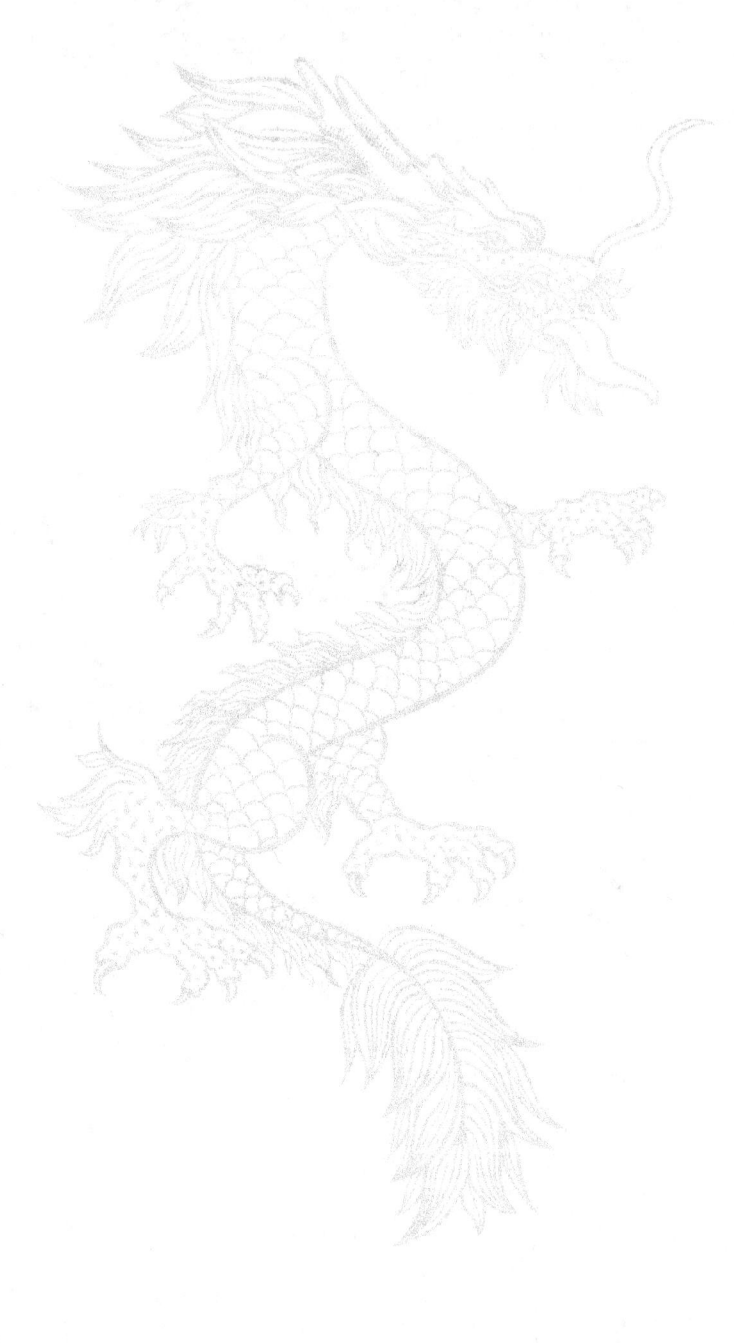

EVERYTHING ZEN

Author's note: *The following short story of Damo (Bodhidharma) is commonly passed down through the different cultural lineages of the Northern and Southern Chinese martial-arts communities. This is my interpretation of his story.*

When the Indian monk Damo climbed down from the mountain above the Shaolin Temple almost fifteen centuries ago, he may have resembled a drifter, but it was eventually learned that his thoughts were majestic. He was obsessively consumed by his life's work to spread his message across the world.

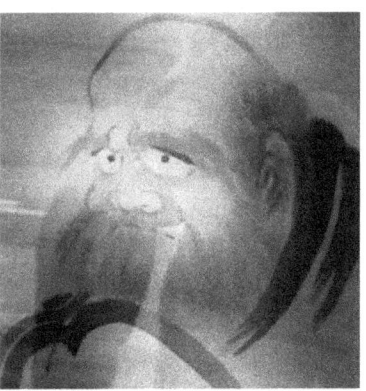

According to legend, Damo received an invitation from the Emperor of China to visit and share his teachings. He traveled from India, crossing many mountains and great rivers across the vast Asian landscape. It was a perilous trek on which he endured many adversities. Nevertheless, his mind was invulnerable and his spirit indomitable. His convictions made his body strong enough to endure. At any time, he could have given up and died on one of those mountains, but his **will** was far too powerful to concede his dream.

Damo looked different from the Chinese. His face was grim with piercing blue eyes and olive skin, his body clothed in a vagabond's rags. Regardless of his appearance, one thing was certain: his heart was possessed with the **determination** to translate his dreams into reality.

Despite being rejected by the emperor and his followers, he continued his journey and stumbled upon the Shaolin Temple where he found his destiny: to become the first patriarch of Zen Buddhism and the refiner of Shaolin martial arts.

ARHAT EXITS THE CAVE

When Damo arrived at the Shaolin Temple, the hospitable monks took him in. It is believed at that time they practiced a form of Hinayana Buddhism. He observed the monk's daily rituals and noticed they possessed terrible personal habits and a poor work ethic. Their training methods were in disarray, lacking the power needed for excellence. There was no system in place and no direction to their practice. They lacked the essential focus for meditation: no connection between the **mind, body, and spirit**. As a result, Damo concluded that their martial arts could be improved if many vital elements were incorporated.

Damo took his ideas and retreated to the nearby mountains to a cave he first observed on his way to the temple. At first, the monks were hesitant to let Damo leave due to his physical condition, but he was insistent. In the cave, he meditated and waited patiently for his creative imagination to kick in. He sat in silence during his vision quest, waiting for instructions.

For nine years, he went back and forth to the cave, devoted to meditation and gazing at the rock wall. Gradually, he developed a renewed purpose in life. Out of that cave came a fire, and almost fifteen centuries later, it is still not extinguished. After nine years, the monks of Shaolin embraced him as their leader.

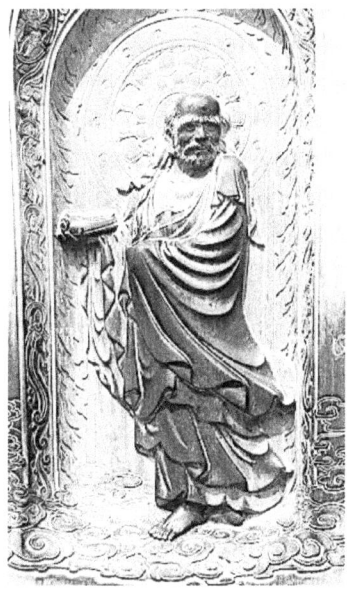

During his vision quest, Damo developed a sophisticated form of philosophy combined with his system of martial arts—now commonly referred to as Zen Buddhism.[1] He invested all of his time, energy, and effort into his life's purpose, and by the end of the decade, a new precedent was set. The beginning of the **Shaolin Warrior** was formed.

With his in-depth knowledge of the internal dynamics of breathing, meditation, yoga, and Indian martial arts, Damo amalgamated these practices to Shaolin kung fu to create the ultimate martial art. This form would invigorate both the internal and external components of the mind, body, and spirit.

As a practice, kung fu encompasses everything that one requires to live a healthy and balanced lifestyle. There are many forms of kung fu, some of which are extravagant and used for exercise, while others are more practical and used for combat. At the time, warriors and bandits from the surrounding countries and areas were often physically bigger and stronger. They commonly defeated Shaolin monks. As a result, the temple would send their men to gather warriors from afar so they could learn different forms of combat to apply to their own techniques. In essence, **kung fu became the original mixed-martial art**. (This form of cross-training or mixing martial arts has existed a lot longer than you might imagine.)

Moving forward, Damo severed ties with his past, renounced the world, and changed his name to Bodhidharma. He unanimously became the twenty-eighth Head Abbot of the Shaolin Temple.[2] Sagacious men and women say, "a leader cannot lead until they know where they are going." So as the leader of the Temple, Bodhidharma traveled to different parts of the Northern and Southern provinces of China to align many of the Buddhist Temples with Zen philosophy. Along the way, he established other Shaolin Temples and spread his Zen teachings across China.

GREAT IMMORTAL SALUTES

The point of the story is this: things may not always happen the way we want them to, but our manifestations will arrive in one form or another—as long as we keep moving forward in carrying out our desires.

In any undertaking, a grasshopper must be willing to sacrifice his entire future. He will forfeit the possibility of retreat if he wishes to reach the enlightened state of mind needed to obtain his desire. There is no retreat, and by no means is there any form of surrender.

It's best to <u>always move forward</u> in any undertaking, especially when fighting for what you want. Even if you must take one step back, follow that with two steps forward. By living your life this way, you will develop the state of mind known as **"the desire to succeed"** which is essential for power.

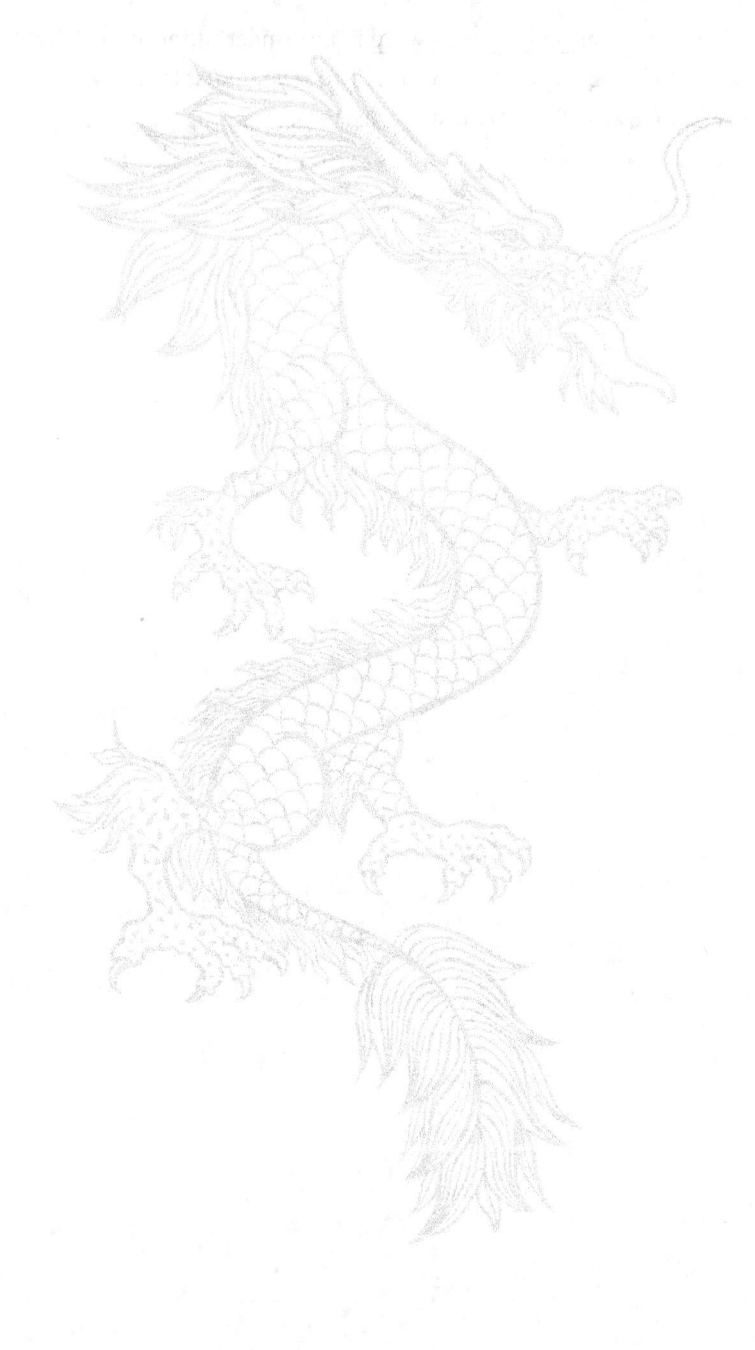

THE ULTIMATE WARRIOR

The samurai were known as "warriors" and served the Emperor of Japan. They followed natural law and the code of *Bushido*, "the way of the warrior." The Bushido Code embodied the characteristics of loyalty, devotion, and honor with an unwavering acceptance of death.[3]

Enter Miyamoto Musashi. Circa 1590, Musashi was a boy who dreamt of becoming a samurai warrior just like his father, Shinmen Munisai. Musashi was born into a family of samurai warriors, and his father was renowned as a great teacher, master of the sword, armor maker, and hand-to-hand combat fighter.

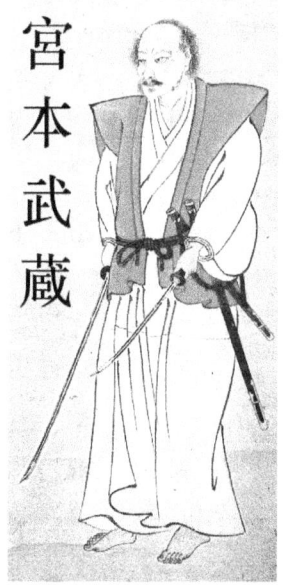

Munisai instilled the philosophies of combat in his son so that Musashi would understand every situation was a matter of life and death—and when someone intended to hurt you, there was no room for error. Consequently, during their father-and-son training sessions, Munisai repeatedly pushed his son to the brink of his physical limits, often injuring Musashi severely in the process.

Musashi perceived this as a form of abuse, and it infused him with deep resentment towards his father. In fact, his father's actions forced Musashi to run away from home at just eight-years-old. However, his ultimate desire to become a samurai never wavered.

THIRTEEN GOING ON ETERNITY

At the age of thirteen, Musashi's life changed forever. A wandering swordsman named Arima who had perfected his skills by engaging in duels across Japan issued a challenge to anyone in Musashi's village. The boy immediately saw an opportunity and accepted the sword fight.

During the duel, Arima made the biggest mistake of his life: he underestimated Musashi because he was just a boy. This ignorance gave Musashi the advantage. He attacked first and struck hard, knocking Arima to the ground, then beating him to a bloody pulp with a wooden staff. Arima's beating was deficient of any skill; it was merely a brutal, psychotic attack that horrified bystanders. At the age of thirteen, Miyamoto Musashi had made his first kill and his desire to become a samurai warrior grew even stronger.

However, Arima's killing left an impression in the villagers' minds, so Musashi's reputation was cast. As a result, he left his village and everything behind, never to return. He made his way to the mountains where he lived and trained in solitude. Nature became his dojo (place for martial arts training).

Without money or armor, he dedicated himself to the discipline of the sword, rising at dawn and spending hour after hour perfecting his skills. He developed a unique two-sword killing style, which became his specialty. The two-sword style took him over forty years to perfect, nevertheless his mastery of the style made him *invincible.*

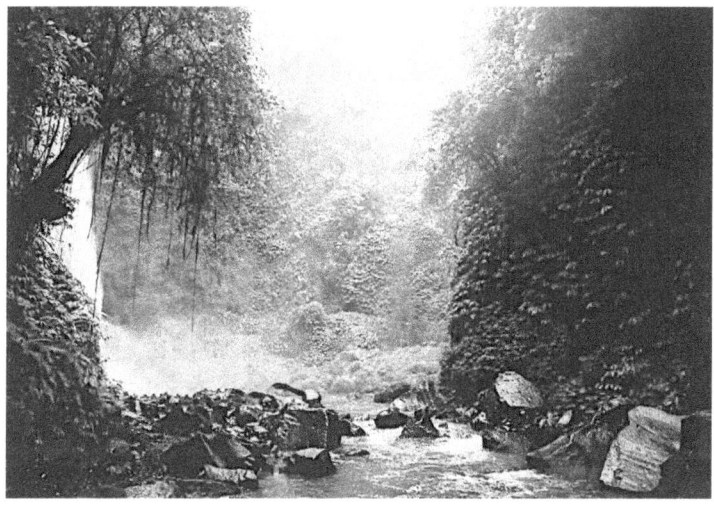

After four years of rigorous training, self-discipline, and solitude in the mountains, Musashi emerged from the wilderness as a skilled warrior. He engaged in another duel, which he won with conviction. Then, at seventeen, he took part in a battle to become an official samurai of the Emperor Go-Yōzei. Although he was on the losing side and almost lost his life, he gained the experience of a lifetime.

THE BATTLE OF SEKIGAHARA

Musashi's first wartime experience was on one of the bloodiest battlefields in Japan's history, the Battle of Sekigahara. Over 160,000 samurai fought and more than 80,000 died in a single day. After the battle, any survivors were killed on sight, but Musashi managed to escape. He made his way back to the wilderness and became a *Ronin*, a "masterless samurai." During this period of feudal Japan, there were many wandering samurai warriors who fell into this category.[4]

The Battle of Sekigahara made Musashi recognize something important: to be a samurai warrior, he would have to become a killing machine—always clenching his fists and gripping his weapon girded by the thought of killing. The battle enhanced his cunning grasp of psychology in combat and led him to further his practices with a darker mindset.

Musashi never forgot that he could die at any time. He remembered this daily, and it made him appreciate life's preciousness. He trained even harder than before. At this time, he also started to think pragmatically. He recognized that **conditioning** and **flexibility** were important for combat, and this allowed him to be more fluid in his technique. He also realized that martial arts are perishable skills—that is, if you don't practice them every day, you will lose them.

SHOGUN'S ASSASSIN

Eventually, Musashi made his way back to the competition circuit where he won duel after duel using psychological tactics: studying his opponents, their weapons, and their habitual tendencies. He became infamous throughout Japan as a master of psychological warfare (i.e. mind games).

In 1612, his most significant victory came when he dueled with the Shogun's martial-arts teacher, Sasaki Kojiro. Musashi knew that if he went to Kyoto and beat the master of one of the most famous sword schools in Japan, he would become an overnight legend.

Musashi thoroughly researched his opponent and noticed that Kojiro's sword was always longer than his opponent's. By making his weapon a little longer than Kojiro's, Musashi gained the needed advantage to win.

He never lost a sword fight, becoming the greatest swordsman of all time, winning over sixty duels. His death in 1645 is believed to be from lung cancer. To this day, Musashi is celebrated in Japan—he even has a railway station named after him. His incredible sense of lifelong dedication and his focus on following the path of the samurai warrior never faltered.

What's more, his philosophies are still studied by educational institutions and business schools throughout Japan and the rest of the world. *TIME Magazine* once wrote, *"On Wall Street, when Musashi speaks, people listen."*[5]

Musashi's experience and wisdom show us what it takes to have dedication and it all starts with a **burning desire and faith**. Any routine or technique (whether it's in martial arts, school, business, sports, or relationships) must be **precise**. <u>You must always think and act in a certain way to achieve success.</u>

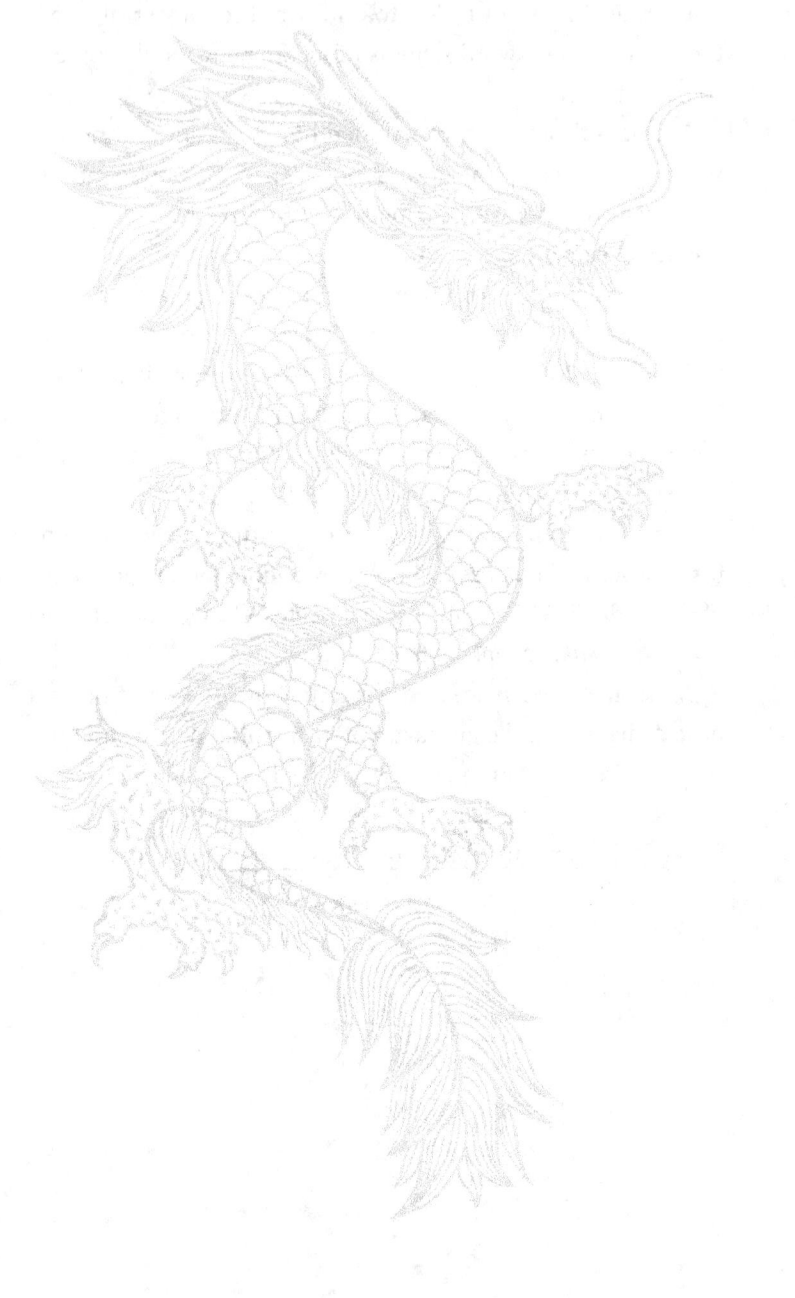

THE LITTLE DRAGON TAKES FLIGHT

In 1959, Bruce Lee set sail from Hong Kong to the United States, which many at the time regarded as "the land of golden opportunity." The most important carry-on item in his possession was his desire to be the **face of greatness**.

Behind him was a tumultuous time in Hong Kong's history, and Lee had experienced a tough time staying out of mischief. He was always in trouble and getting into fights with bullies. His parents agreed that he would join a martial-arts academy run by the famous master Ip Man who would teach Lee the fundamentals of Wing Chun kung fu. Although this training was short-lived, Ip Man's teachings helped shape Lee into a man who commanded respect and admiration from the world.[6]

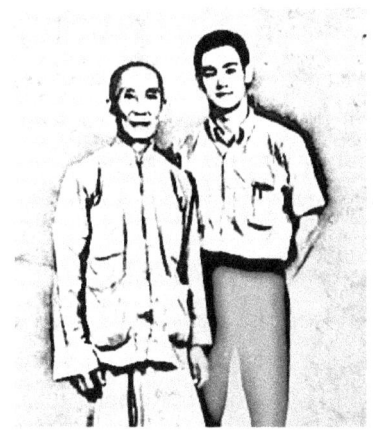

The chance for a new start in the land of golden opportunity meant unlimited potential for Lee, who had an ambitious heart and a thirst for success. His desire for greatness helped him create an epic destiny that continues almost fifty years after his death.

In San Francisco, Lee pursued his training by learning a northern style of Shaolin kung fu taught by his uncle. He traded dance lessons for martial arts, perfecting his movement and footwork in both dancing and combat.

Eventually, Lee moved to Washington State where he enrolled in the University of Seattle. He studied philosophy, which intensified his interest in the difference between Eastern and Western cultures, and the philosophical teachings behind martial arts and success.

At college, Lee established a martial-arts school for students on campus. He offered classes including strenuous conditioning exercises, self-defense applications, and combat sparring. He combined Eastern Chinese disciplines with his creative imagination to revolutionize martial arts—forging a new philosophy of reality-based fighting and martial arts combat that wasn't restricted by fixed patterns, like other existing martial arts styles.

WAY OF THE INTERCEPTING FIST

In 1964, Lee married and relocated from Washington State to California, but his desire to spread his martial arts philosophy didn't fade. He teamed up with martial-arts expert James Yimm Lee and together they opened Bruce Lee's second martial arts school in Oakland.

At the time, Bruce Lee had become enemies with the rival martial-arts schools in the area. The masters of these schools issued a challenge for Lee to fight a young teacher from Hong Kong, Wong Jack Man, who had a school in San Francisco.

This fight changed Lee's perspective on the concept of martial arts altogether. After recognizing his weaknesses, he began experimenting with various martial arts, adopting a variety of techniques from Wing Chun, Filipino martial arts, judo, savate, boxing, and fencing to create a new style of fighting called *Jeet Kune Do*. In Cantonese, it translates as **"the way of the intercepting fist."**[7]

Lee's theory was that to be successful in combat, the techniques used during a fight must be improvised and not bound by the traditions of form or routine. He felt so passionate about his new martial-arts style that he opened another school in Los Angeles with fellow martial-arts practitioner Dan Inosanto, at which point he started to reach the pinnacle of his training.

MAN, MYTH, LEGEND

At the same time, Lee was a martial-arts teacher for several Hollywood movie stars who enticed him to take up acting. After accruing several small roles, his career began to change. Despite having multiple schools open, he wanted to share his new philosophy and martial arts style with the wider world.

The conflict between establishing a national chain of martial-arts schools and pursuing an acting career wore heavily on him. After thorough self-reflection, he realized that his vision would reach more people through film, and this burning desire left an iconic imprint on the world.

To fulfill his ultimate destiny, Lee sacrificed himself. He left everything behind—his family, his country, and even life itself. Before his death, he went back to Hong Kong and filmed several critically acclaimed box office hits including *The Big Boss*,[8] *Fist of Fury*,[9] and *Way of the Dragon*.[10] Finally, when he made *Enter the Dragon* with Warner Bros.,[11] he reached worldwide success. However, by the time it was released, Lee had died from a cerebral edema, and he never got the chance to experience the global recognition that his movie received.

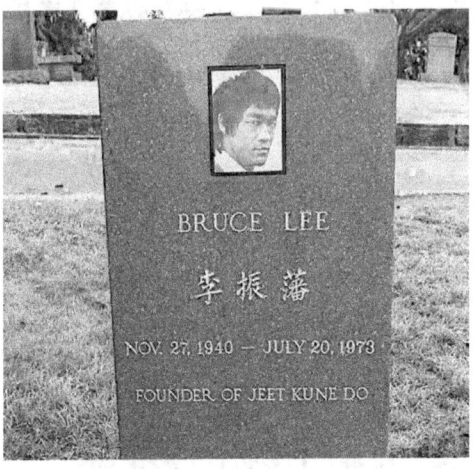

Note: *Bruce Lee's son, Brandon, died suddenly and tragically while filming the movie "The Crow."*[12] *For those who grew up on Bruce Lee films, the death of Brandon Lee drew a similar intrigue and mystique, due to his death while filming such an iconic unfinished role, which felt meaningful and ominous.*

Over 25,000 people attended Bruce Lee's funeral and flooded the streets of Hong Kong. It's reported that over 100,000 people visit his grave annually in Seattle, a remarkable illustration of his impact on the world.[13] Lee's legacy is not only being one of the greatest martial artists to have ever lived, but also being the father of modern-day mixed martial arts.

I now embrace the world and step out on the true path.

To live, learn, and attain truth for light and love.

My worldly cares are gone, and in return I have grace.

I vow to help all, so they may also see the way.

— Zen Mantra

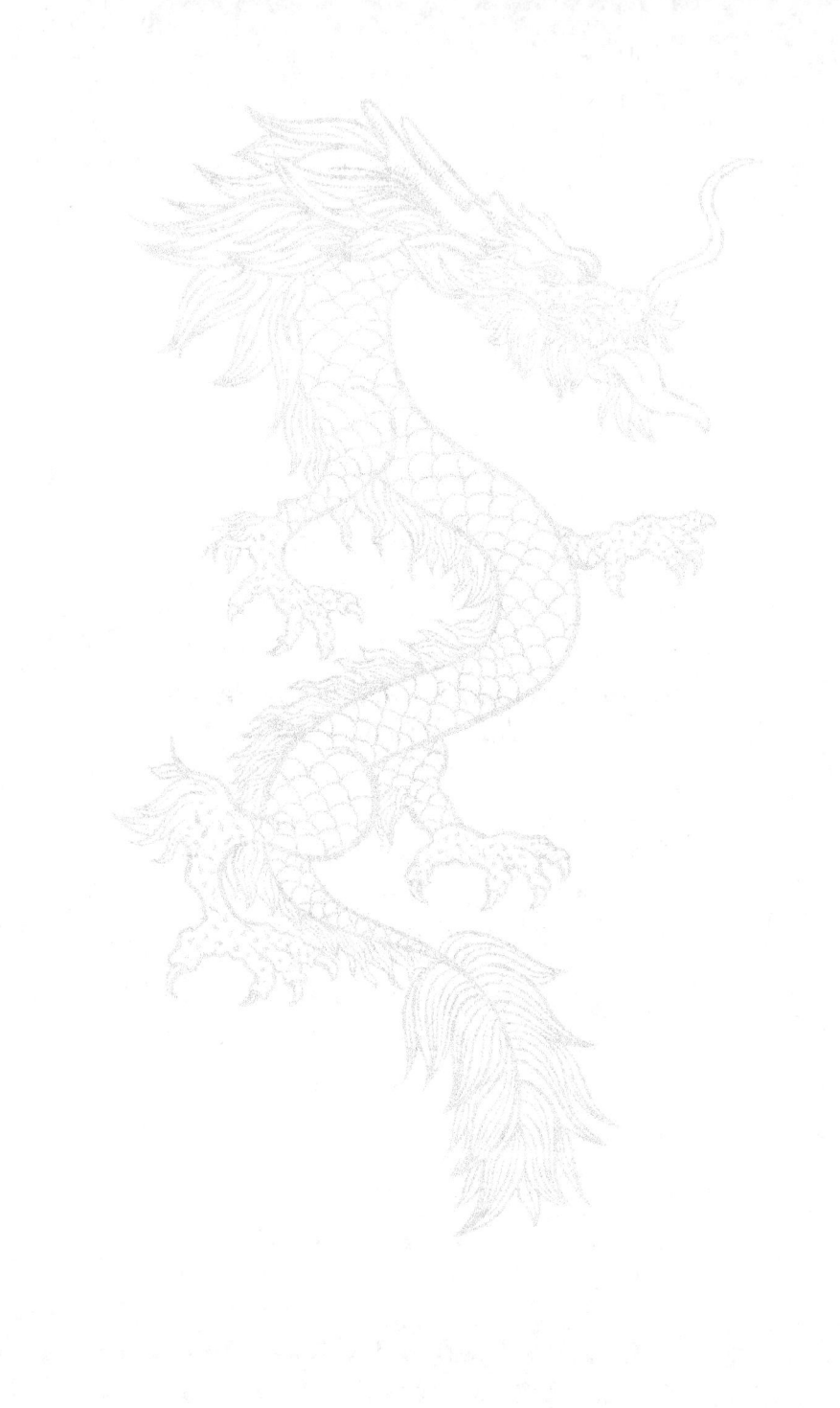

INTRODUCTION

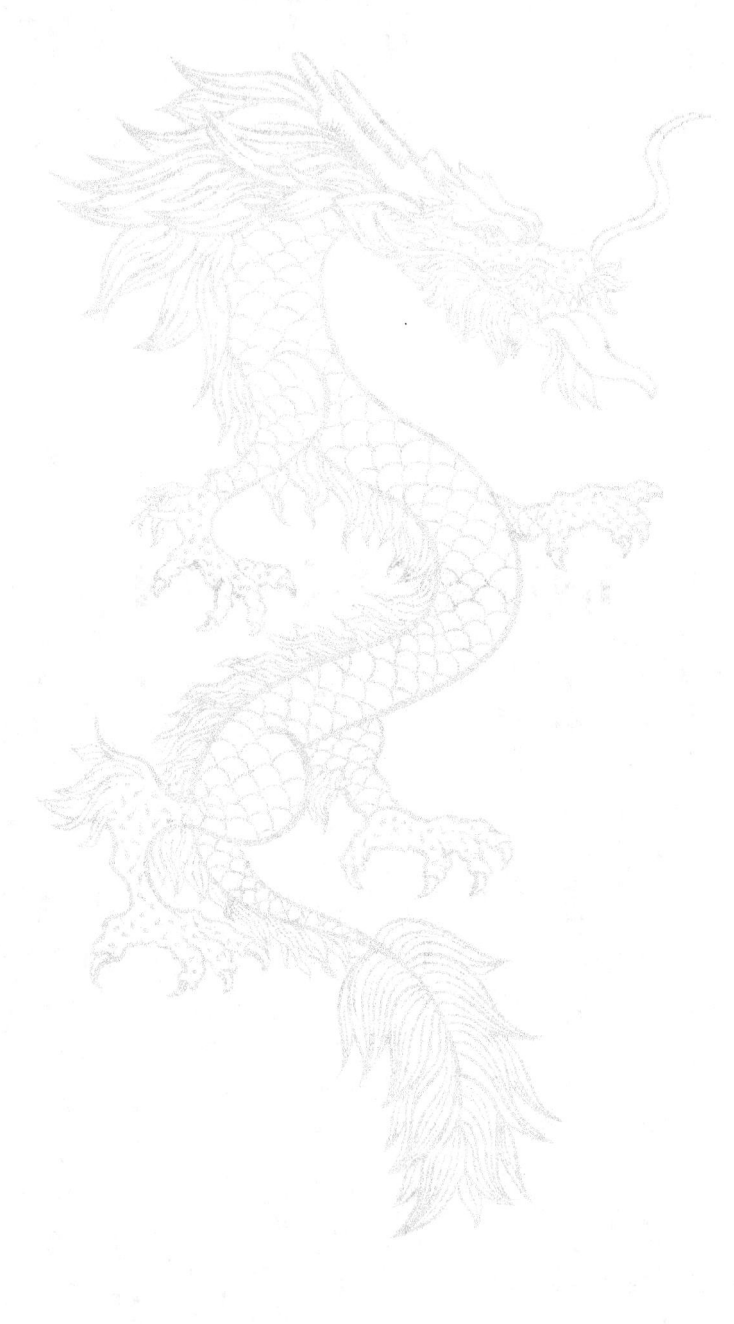

THE POWER WITHIN YOU

We are all born with a link to invincible power. Somewhere down the line, we lose our connection to this power by inheriting the ways of our well-meaning parents, teachers, and friends who impose their limitations upon us. As a result, these limitations program us into believing what we can and cannot do. Those who shield themselves from these limiting beliefs by developing mental strength and a healthy body can create a life beyond boundaries.

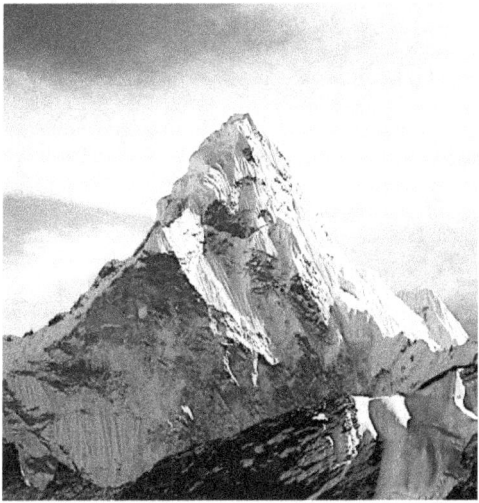

Every day, there are unbelievable great feats performed by ordinary men and women across all walks of life. This book will show you how these feats are possible.

It's true that what one man or woman can do, another can do; however, some men and women have the gift of creating or doing something *never done before*. Sir Edmund Hillary[14] did "the impossible" when he climbed Mt. Everest in 1953—and thousands of men and women have followed in his footsteps. Sir Hillary was told by his friends and family not to go because he would die on the mountain. Instead, he conquered Mt. Everest.

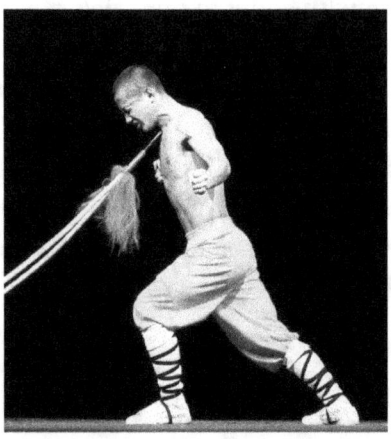

Some people can walk on hot coals. Others can elevate their internal heat during freezing temperatures while wearing a wet towel on their back. I have witnessed men take a spear to the throat without it piercing the skin, and others take a powerful kick to the groin without flinching. Most things are possible when you set your mind to it.

It is my belief that human beings are the highest form of creation for a reason, and we must keep this in mind during every thought impulse and before every action we take in life.

Every one of us can quickly become a slave to external conditions and the negative circumstances of life. To resolve this, we often seek strength from an outside source, yet all the power we genuinely need comes from within ourselves. This power makes us who we are, and we must unfold and develop this as we progress through our lives.

THE PATH TO POWER

The path to power consists of **growth, development,** and **self-control.** A disciplined mind forges a healthy body, and together they establish an indomitable spirit. This spirit is the purpose of this book. *We all have the spirit to become, to be, and to do whatever we want.*

This book will help you better understand yourself, and assist in raising your **spiritual vibration**[*] to reach a higher level of martial arts. Unfortunately, many people have rigid beliefs, and mock spirituality as something mystical or delusional, which isn't the case. In this book, I hope to bring a greater understanding to the *practical* sense of spirituality for anyone who remains cynical.

Through the ages, spirituality is what kept humans alive and assisted our survival. It's essential to understand how you as a person, warrior, or spiritual being has evolved through the ages into this modern world—and how the best version of you can be brought about to serve others and help you reach the ultimate goal in life: *a link to infinite power.*

If you don't know who you are, what you are, what you want, and where you want to be, this book will serve as a guide to find your truth. It's not difficult to figure these things out—you just have to be willing to invest the time to look deep within yourself.

I write this book with no ego, as if I were writing to myself when I was younger, ignorant, and ultimately lost, so it's designed to help you find your way on to the right path. Let this book

---

[*] Your thoughts and actions create vibrations in the world's external etheric energy fields. Your spiritual vibration is your energy force that makes an imprint or difference in the external world.

serve you and assist you in finding the **power within you**. It all begins with a desire.

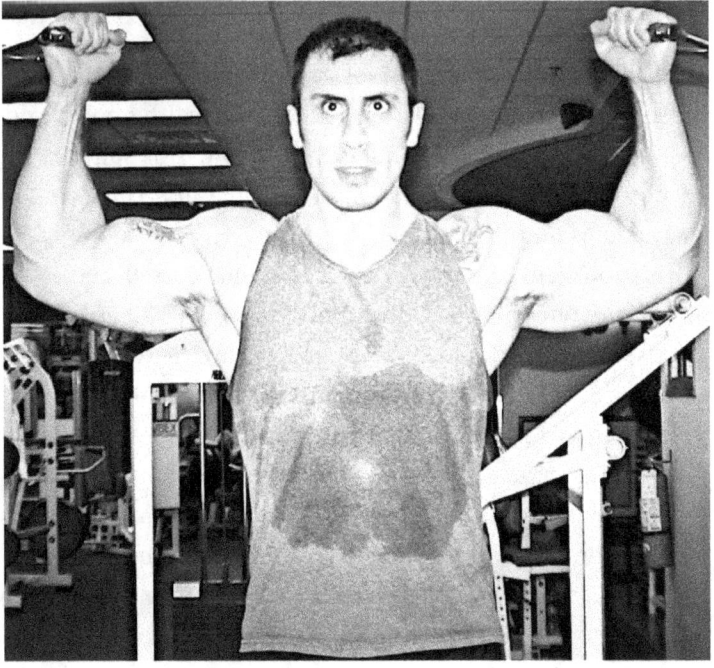

WHAT IS INVINCIBILITY?

Perhaps you're reading this book because you're captivated by invincibility? I too have always been obsessed with invincibility. This quality is the goal of most martial artists, however, the true nature of invincibility is often misconstrued.

Invincibility isn't limited to feeling no pain or becoming bulletproof, it has many facets. The true essence of invincibility is *infinite*. Please understand that when I use the word "invincible," it is not meant to fool you. It doesn't mean that if you read this book, you will become impervious to pain, never die, or any other outrageous claim. What's more, my definition of invincibility may be different from yours, and the outcome of each power obtained might vary.

To differentiate fact from fiction through the practices I outline in this book, you can optimize the physical and mental conditions needed to look and feel *invincible*.

The true power of invincibility is **freedom**, a belief that can be tapped into at any time to embrace your vulnerabilities, overcome obstacles, and fulfill your needs. It is about feeling pain, embracing it, appreciating it, and realizing that it is there to challenge you to become your best and thereby overcome the pain.

This book will stimulate your mind, help revitalize your body, and invigorate your soul. I wrote it to help you through all aspects in life, not just martial arts. This book can be your guide or teacher—something that you can come back to at any time in your life to help you on your journey.

I wish it were simple to convey the journey towards invincibility in the quickest and shortest way possible. To give you the complete picture, take your discovery step by step. With each lesson in this book, take the time to digest it, meditate on it, and allow it to unfold the power within you. (Don't worry if you don't yet know how to meditate, as you will learn how.)

This whole philosophy will take time, and yet it is time that will shape you accordingly. Be patient, and don't rush, only arrogant fools rush in to the unknown. Keep your thoughts majestic like Bodhidharma. When you finally arrive at your destination, you will keep everything you have earned and be king of the mountain for as long as you wish.

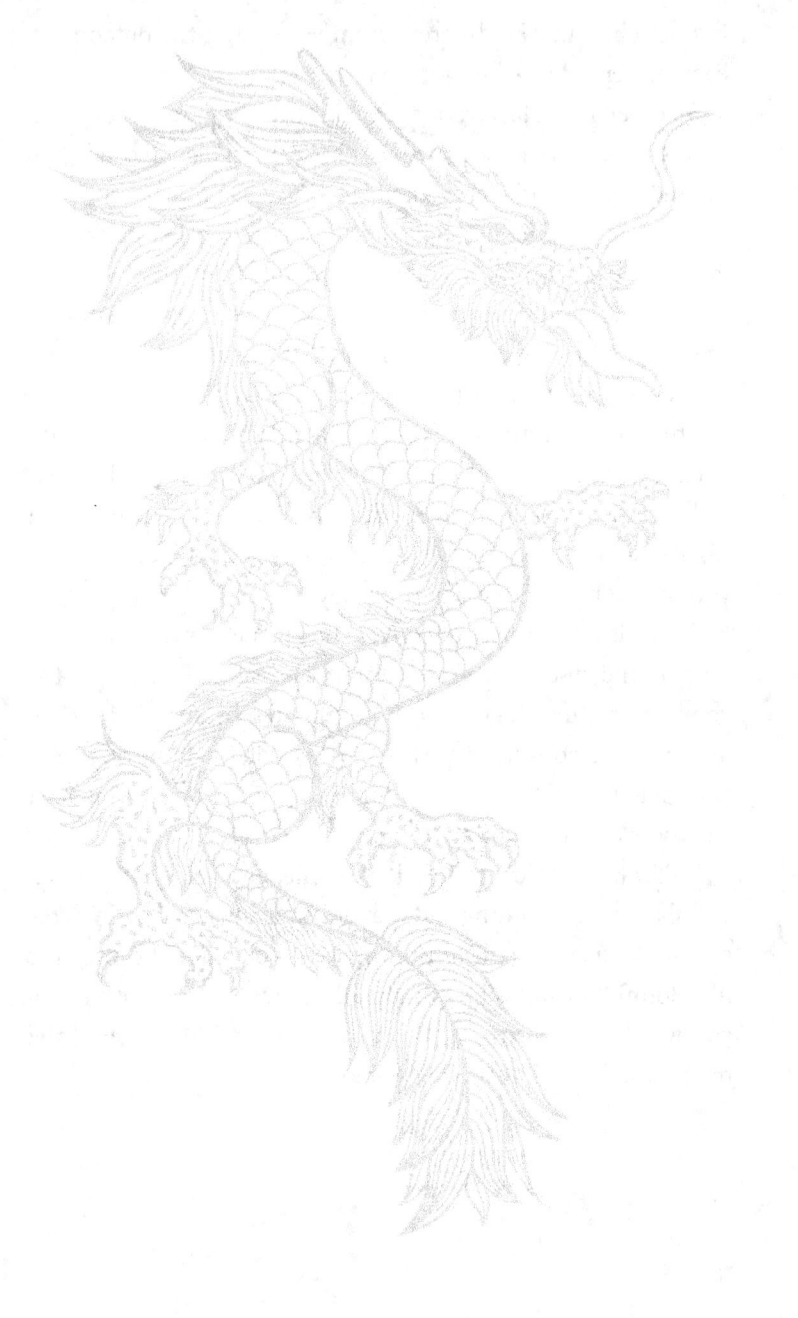

POWER-CONSCIOUSNESS

The basis of this book is to help you acquire **power**. You may find it challenging to understand all of it, or even agree with it, and that's fine. However, it will assist you in one way or another. Each chapter is a lesson with objectives to absorb and apply. These lessons will help you plant the seeds to grow the power you seek. The development and application of power is threefold:
1. PHYSICAL: The amount of strength applied in the shortest amount of time.
2. MENTAL: Knowledge organized and intelligently directed towards a specific purpose.
3. SPIRITUAL: The effectiveness of applied faith in everything you do.

Power is an idea that we can convert into reality. However, most of the time it remains dormant unless it's cultivated and applied through action or practice. We blend vital energy to obtain power with the following four principles:
1. MOTIVE: An intense burning **desire** for power or a specific purpose.
2. BELIEF: The **faith** in oneself, other people, and a higher power.
3. PLAN: The organization of **knowledge**.
4. PERSISTENCE: The relentless tenacity to follow through with plans.

The motive behind any purpose must be **authentic**. This energy—through the physical, mental, and spiritual gates—provides your overall level of **power-consciousness**. But to acquire power, you have to keep practicing in all three areas. This trinity is ultimately called the **mind-body-spirit connection**, and it's necessary for the gift or treasure that is the focal point of this book.

We all need power in life, whether it is physical, mental, or spiritual. In the physical sense, we attain power through the methods found in martial arts, fitness, conditioning, and cultivating our internal energy. This book discusses all of these methods.

A connection to infinite power is difficult when you're unaware that the connection exists. Power-consciousness helps us recognize that we can achieve anything in life. With this awareness, life has a deeper, fuller meaning. You see things more clearly and appreciate that all of your hopes and dreams may come true. As clichéd as that sounds, <u>you learn by going within</u>, and the more you know about yourself, the more you can be in control of your life.

You have absolute control over your thoughts, choices, and actions. This gift is so significant for all men, women, and children. To gain power-consciousness, there can be no fears, worries, doubts, or indecision, because these destructive thoughts are harmful and can subdue the power within you.

One of the essential steps to procure power-consciousness is preparing your mind for the attainment of your desire. This process will be your greatest challenge and will determine whether you can absorb this philosophy. The best way to learn who you are or what you can accomplish is by <u>first knowing what you desire</u>.

Power-consciousness is a state of mind that you must create. You cannot buy it for any price. Keep your state of mind impenetrable to weakness, there is no other way to success. This book is your guide on the path to power. If you neglect the journey or stop before you arrive, you have no one to blame but yourself. There are no excuses that can save you. Accept responsibility for your life and take control.

To acquire power, we must not remain static, but keep learning, developing, and growing. Any skill without effectiveness is empty, so your force must endure the process of growth and development to become powerful.

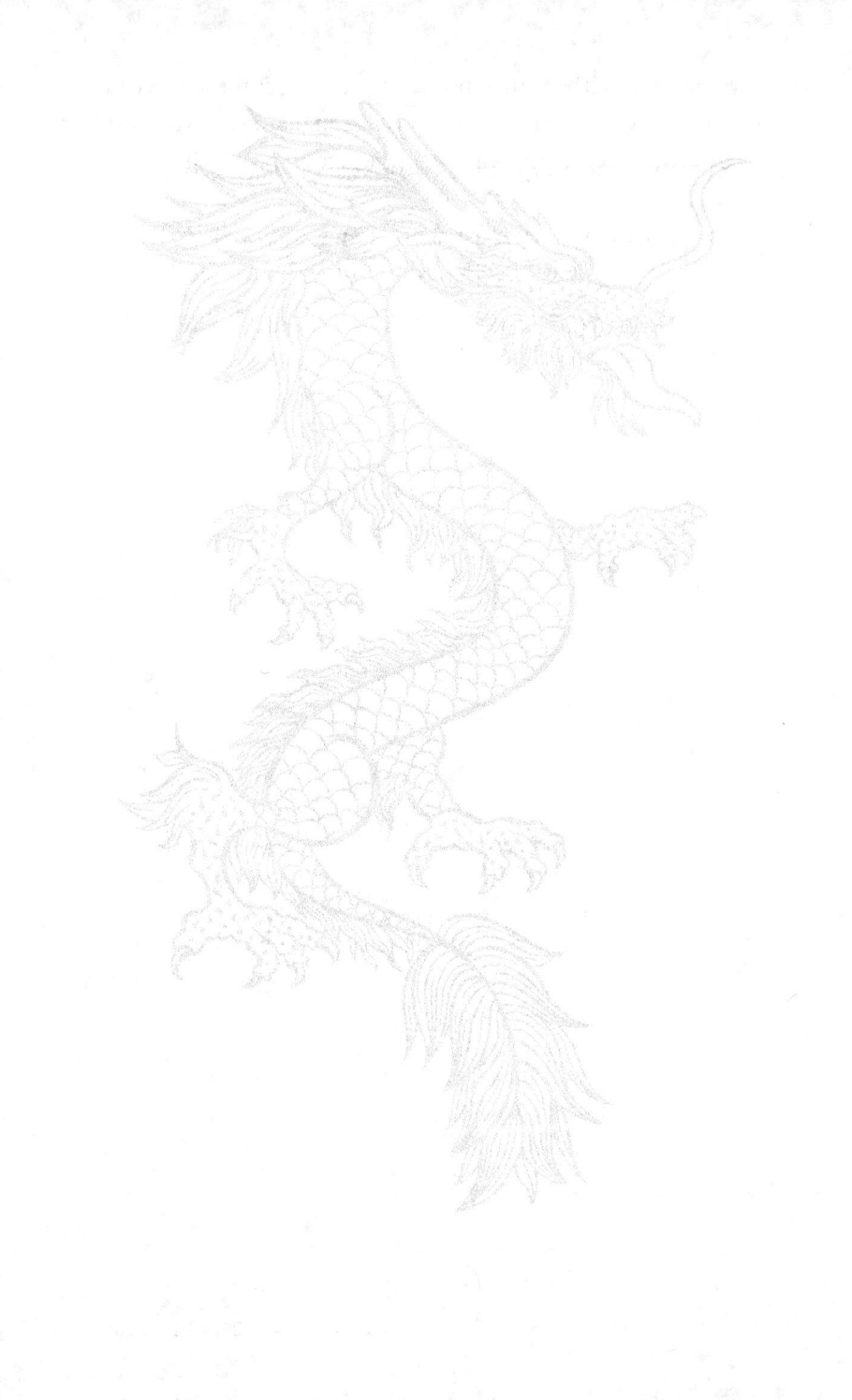

THE MOTIVE DRIVES POWER

When driven by a motive that becomes an obsession, any man or woman is capable of remarkable achievements. However, to achieve power, they must be willing to change their **mindset** and **habits**.

If you wish to control your life and harness the power within, take control of your mind when it's in action. <u>If you do not control your mind, someone or something else might</u>. Your thoughts are significant because they are the key to your power-consciousness and they monitor your body.

Constructive thoughts and positive emotions must dominate your mind. This means you need to eliminate the negative emotions or petty annoyances that you encounter on a daily basis. Remember that life is full of ups and downs—they are simply like changing degrees in temperature, and you have to practice acceptance.

The good news is that anything your mind can conceive, your body can achieve. It all starts with having **mind control**, which is the result of self-discipline through daily habits. We humans are creatures of habit, and we discipline our actions towards betterment through **service, training, nutrition,** and **meditation**.

The power to control our habits develops through the force of **willpower,** and habitual persistence creates discipline that controls the mind.

To convert the desire for power into physical reality, follow the path that I have laid out before you. If you exercise self-control and direct it towards the attainment of power, your success is within reach.

THE NINE GATES TO INVINCIBILITY

The method to transform power into physical reality involves nine basic principles or **gates**. You will pass the first three gates in this book, and when you are ready, you can move on to the following three gates, which you will find in my next book, and the final three gates in the third volume.

The first gate is "dedication to a specific purpose." This could be martial arts, a sport, a musical instrument, or even schoolwork. For me, this was martial arts—it is what got me to this point in my life. I felt that our world needed a practical, understandable philosophy for martial artists looking to connect their mind-body-spirit to achieve greatness. As you are reading this book, I assume that martial arts are likely also your purpose, but the lessons within this book can also be applied to other purposes.

The Nine Gates to Invincibility are not just about achieving invulnerability, but achieving success in every aspect of life. This book is a guide to obtaining power, and each gate can help you acquire whatever you desire in life.

However, it will only work if you <u>believe and have faith in yourself</u>, and continue to practice your actions with due diligence, even if it takes the rest of your life. Remember the three warriors from the preface?

1. **Bodhidharma** achieved invincibility because of his iron-clad willpower, and as a result, he became the leader of the Shaolin Temple and the first patriarch of Zen Buddhism.

2. **Miyamoto Musashi** achieved invincibility because of his unwavering focus, courage, discipline, and persistence, and he became the greatest swordsman who ever lived.
3. **Bruce Lee** attained invincibility because he constantly strived for betterment without limitations, and he became a legend.

So, how can you understand and harness the power within this book? The answer is within you, though the pages before you act as a guide. Each section alone is not sufficient to attain power, but the book as a whole has the answer. At the end, a whole new reality will reveal itself to you.

THE GRASSHOPPER

"The grasshopper" is what you are when you first start your journey. At first, the grasshopper is unfaithful to anything and bounces around from person to person, place to place, and object to object. It lacks confidence, has no regard for others, and has no faith in anything, including itself. In essence, the grasshopper is an insect with no spirit.

Your **spirit** is vital, and its central principle is that all power comes from within you. This power that you hold is spiritual, and all spirit is one. Everything is part of the whole. This recognition and acceptance will bring about all of the conditions in your life that align with your purpose.

Most human beings develop what is called "the grasshopper mentality,"[15] which means a mind that jumps from one thing to another, never sticking around long enough to fully benefit from any concept. Grasshoppers are full of thoughts and ideas, but never see any of them through to completion.

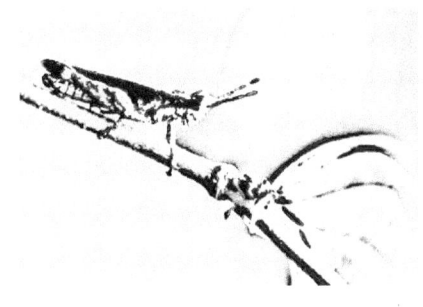

The grasshopper observes too much and retains too little. It forms destructive habits, influenced by its surroundings and other people's opinions. It develops an inability to be creative and organize plans, because its focal point is always on its surroundings and fellow grasshoppers, never on itself or the task at hand.

The solution to all of the grasshopper's problems and prayers is to learn **the art of concentrated thought,** which is not just a benefit in martial arts, but in life. If the grasshopper tamed all of its desires into one specific purpose, it would open the gate to obtain treasures in every area of life. Unfortunately, its mentality doesn't allow it to stay focused for long enough, and so the grasshopper remains undisciplined, and its thoughts flow with the wind.

Concentrated thought is deeply related to certainty of purpose. However, it also requires self-determination, and this has a price—one that the grasshopper pays if it wants to evolve. Its evolution can lead to power—if only it can concentrate long enough to remain focused.

While the grasshopper jumps from object to object, the warrior stays committed to a purpose and connected to the inner spirit indefinitely. Commitment is an essential characteristic of life. This is how you live—committed to everything that you are and everything that you do.

And now, to the first gate. . . .

GATE 1—
MARTIAL ARTS

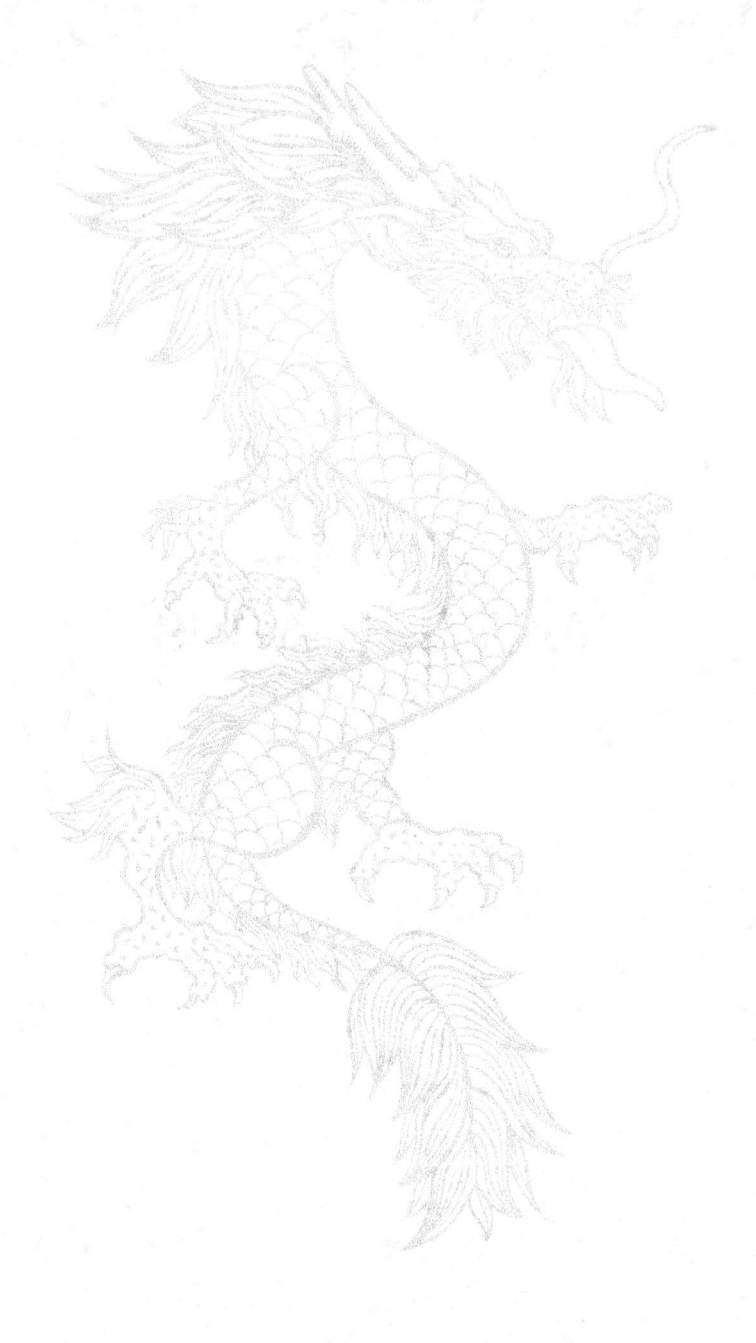

GATEWAY TO THE TEMPLE OF DESIRE

Welcome to the first gate, the starting point towards invincibility. For me, this gateway to the temple of desire opened when I found my purpose, and that is when I began to tap into my most significant potential in life.

Before learning better, I lived in a material world driven by my false ego, always seeking power externally. I was a grasshopper and bounced around with no direction or purpose.

Earl Nightingale said: *"A man without a plan is like a ship without a course. With no place to go, disaster is a probability."*[16]

Thomas Carlyle stated: *"A man without a purpose is like a ship without a rudder—a waif, a nothing, a no man."*[17]

I was living proof of these two statements. Everybody needs a purpose in life, something they can use to express themselves physically, mentally, and spiritually.

Over the years, I devoted myself to rigorous physical training and continuously got lost in mental anguish. It wasn't until I tapped into the power within me that I brought a whole new existence into my perception, and it led me to my life's purpose.

Martial arts are unique because they strengthen our minds. The **conscious mind** is our link to the outside world and it allows us to connect physically and emotionally. The conscious mind is a guardian to the inner thoughts, ideas, and experiences that may imprint the subconscious mind, and when we have control of our minds, we become stronger within.

Through martial arts, I developed a passion for practicing diligently to perfect my techniques. The same obsession is in the blood of every true martial artist. As time passes, we gain more inspiration, we build momentum, and our spirit enhances. We become conscious that there is no such thing as "something for nothing." Everything I ever desired in life had a price, and I had to pay that price for my plans or wishes to materialize. The price for any martial artist is a lifetime of devoted practice.

THE LIFE-CHANGER

I grew up in a tumultuous environment dominated by negativity. Before adopting martial arts into my life, I had no direction or self-worth. I had no respect for others or for myself, but when I started to delve deep into my training, my spirit evoked a transformation.

Thankfully, I grew from an anxious, fearful boy into a strong, confident, successful man. Martial arts taught me so much about the ways of the world and how to be a better man. They gave me the knowledge, wisdom, and self-discipline to live a life of purpose, direction, and fulfillment.

Thanks to martial arts, I have:

- Learned how to cultivate order in my life and live it the way I want.
- Attracted positive people and circumstances into my life that are in harmony with my purpose.
- Started a successful business from scratch and learned how to put people first by applying the golden rule,† helping them change for the better. By helping others win, I end up winning as well, bringing positive energy into every area of my life.
- Opened a gateway to a life that has brought me treasures: excellent health, love, friendships, happiness, positive

---

† The biblical rule, "do to others as you would have them do to you." (Luke 6:31, NIV)

energy, wisdom, power, strength, courage, self-confidence, and success.
- Learned how to put my ego aside and embrace love for the first time, from a good woman who has supported me throughout all of my frustrations and all of my successes.
- Faith in my fellow man, a higher loving power, and myself—something I never had when I was growing up.

In addition, martial arts not only enhanced my life but saved my life as well. We all go through hardships and struggles, but I'm here to tell you that you can overcome them. Martial arts have been that constant factor in my life helping me overcome any challenge I have faced. When fear, pain, anxiety, paranoia, indecision, superstition, doubt, poverty, loss, or heartbreak tries to master me, my training helps carry me over the top and win every single time.

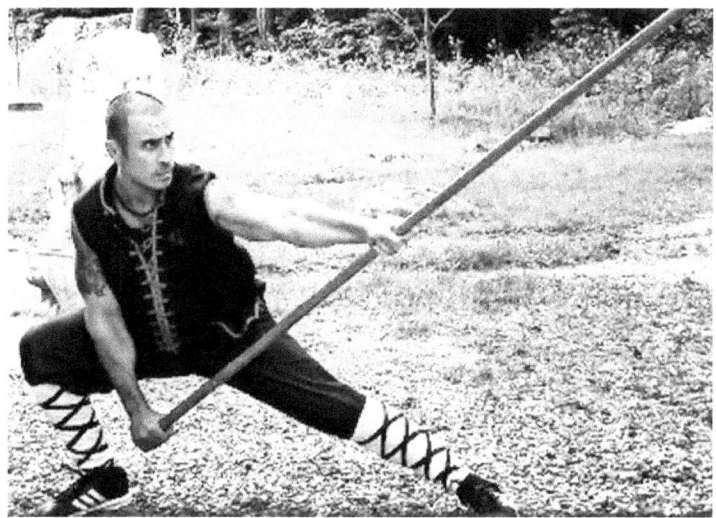

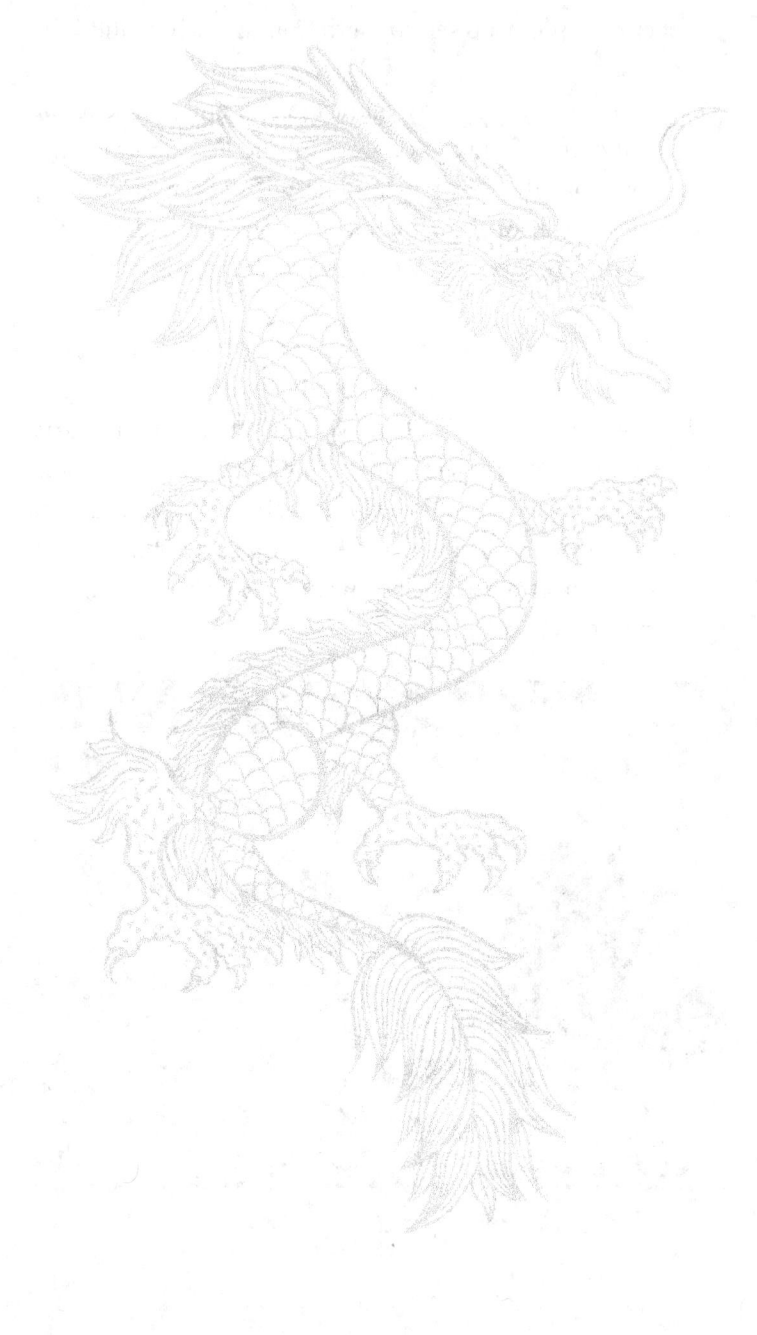

CHAPTER 1: WHAT ARE MARTIAL ARTS?

Most martial arts derive from Chinese kung fu, which summons the essences of **animal spirits** within you and employs the **five elements** (earth, fire, water, metal, and wood) to express them. Anyone can learn martial arts and practice their techniques by performing the movements with their hands and feet, but the animal spirit behind each action and the elements that deliver them are what makes you powerful.

The same way that a musician learns an instrument or an artist discovers how to use a paintbrush, martial arts teach you how to connect with nature and other human beings using the animal and element techniques.

These components become an extension of you in your daily activities.

Over the years, I have found that martial arts are essential in life for many reasons:

- Firstly, you need to know how to defend yourself, as self-defense is a vital attribute at any age. Not knowing how to protect yourself is a weakness you cannot afford.
- Secondly, martial arts enable you to develop skills that are gateways to conquering the flaws within you.
- Finally, they build confidence, giving you unwavering courage toward any action, and helping you to overcome your fears and obstacles.

Martial arts induce the warrior within you, and they enable an individual's inner light to shine brightly from their solar plexus, becoming a source of strength and courage for others. This light radiates as brightly as the sun, bringing warmth and comfort to those around you who are suffering or looking for security. The individual also becomes attractive and magnetic.

Whoever you are, whatever you do, martial arts enable you to prepare for conflicts that arise in your life. Although conflict is essential to your growth and development, martial arts provide you with the tools, energy, awareness, and attitude to overcome challenges, because they help cultivate growth from within.

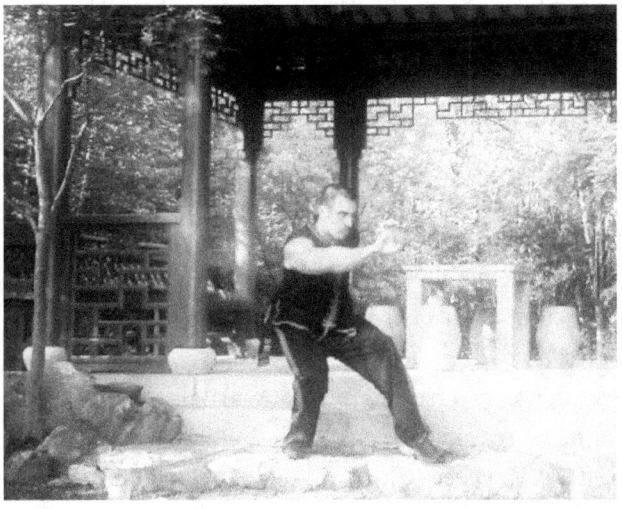

For most practitioners, the grasshopper mindset understands martial arts techniques as some form of fighting ability that can make you superior to your opponent. This form of thinking is where growth begins, and it becomes your mental conception of power.

After many years of training, the grasshopper hopefully learns that martial arts aren't just physical, but also mental and spiritual.

Some are attracted to these aspects of training, others are not. Although martial arts might not be the "be all, end all" for everybody, its philosophies will help to cultivate the power that comes from within you.

Most people get distracted easily, and the majority will quit before they achieve their desires. Yet, it's far better if you persist in your practice until your dying breath—no matter what. You develop power through purpose, and if you train hard enough and keep adjusting your form, practice eventually makes perfect. You become who you want to be and obtain what you want to have.

FOUR FINGERS HOLD UP THE SKY

Whether it's biology, chemistry, or physics, each plays a crucial role in helping human beings understand life. Science is the study of the behavior and structure of both the physical and the natural world through observation and experimentation. When you consider the depth of the subject and the different fields within it, it's apparent that the study never ends. The same goes for martial arts since it is an internal and external science related to the cultivation and expression of energy.

1. **Internal science of martial arts:** How the body produces and uses internal energy for wellbeing and well-doing.
2. **External science of martial arts:** How the mind and body act and react to objective situations with external expressions of energy.

The time and effort you apply to both observation and experimentation can lead to many useful results. In martial arts, the study and practice never ends.

A wealth of information has contributed to the attainment of knowledge throughout the ages. Whenever you try to better yourself in any manner, you gain more understanding, clarity, and depth of vision. When we dedicate our thoughts to following an organized plan through persistent action, we receive the power we seek. Earning these skills will improve your spiritual growth, which is necessary to attain power-consciousness.

However, it's challenging to hone your skills. Most people are born, go through life sleepwalking, then they die. They get caught up in the rat race and never gain spiritual growth. They don't think for themselves and instead conform to society's needs, wants, fears, and trends—and their ignorance is passed from one generation to another, never learning that there is no such thing as something for nothing.

Through the study of martial arts, you can learn, teach, heal, and hurt. You can help yourself by helping others, or you can isolate yourself and deny others your gift—the choice is yours. That is the beauty of your training; it can be anything you want it to be. **You are what you create, and you create what you are.**

With this in mind, life takes on a whole new perspective. This ideology allows us to explore ourselves and everything that nature has to offer. You create your life, and what you make of it is your doing. **At any time, you can change anything you want.** The possibilities are endless.

AN INTENSE BURNING DESIRE

In our world, there is soon to be a trillion people and you are one of them, but . . .
- Who are you?
- What makes you unique?
- What do you want to be?
- What do you want to do?
- What do you want to have?

If you don't know the answers to these questions yet, then you'll have trouble cultivating the power within you. The ability to cultivate your power is the thing you'll need to distinguish yourself from everybody else and find your purpose on earth.

To find your purpose, first clarify the vision in your mind. When you're conscious of your **potential power,** it's time to start improving yourself, so you can cultivate that power and express it in alignment with your purpose. To do so, devote yourself towards connecting to your inner spirit. Your spirit helps you forge the desire to pursue your purpose and begin to change your world. Then, everything around you will start falling into place.

This process stems from the **natural law of cause and effect.** The world is the effect and you are the cause. If you want to change any of the results in your life, first address their causes. Then, if you adjust yourself accordingly, new outcomes will stem from that change similar to when you're playing chess or rolling in jiu-jitsu.

Most people wish, want, and crave fulfillment of their desires, but they never follow the blueprint of thinking and acting in a certain way to achieve them. Unfortunately, hoping or wishing for something doesn't mean you will get it. That is a grasshopper's mentality—dealing with effects and hardly ever putting in the effort needed to find the cause or make the necessary changes to produce the desired results.

Grasshoppers force their desires, simultaneously building a resistance to them by subconsciously believing they can never acquire them. Since they never learn the right way to think or act, they burn out or drop out, and never reach attainment. You will always be tested, hijacked, and sabotaged by your ego. But if you truly desire something, never quit reaching.

THE SCIENCE BEHIND SUCCESS

The science behind success principles (*Think & Grow Rich*, Napoleon Hill)[18] is that those who become successful in anything usually devote a significant portion of their thoughts, efforts, and time into becoming the best version of themselves, and preparing and practicing for the achievement of their accomplishments. So to become an influentially successful or powerful person, first have an intense burning obsession, a state of mind that never gives up, and the persistence in following through on all of your plans for achievement.

After studying many of the greats who achieved outstanding success, I have concluded that it was their certainty of purpose to first learn, practice, and better themselves that drove them to their accomplishments. Bodhidharma, Musashi, and Lee are just a few examples of this sacrificial process that embodies the essence of martial arts. This process is beneficial to any human being alive, because it's necessary for anything you're interested in getting better at or achieving.

If you desire to be powerful or successful, develop power-consciousness. To do this, use **visualization**, which helps you see yourself carrying out your purpose or in possession of your desire. Next, practice with the element of fire (i.e. determination). The objective is to become so determined to perfect your skills that you start becoming the best version of yourself.

Allow your mind to become so thoroughly saturated with the vision of attainment, practice, and your progress that you can already see yourself possessing what you seek. This gift of idealization, visualization, and action are available to everyone.

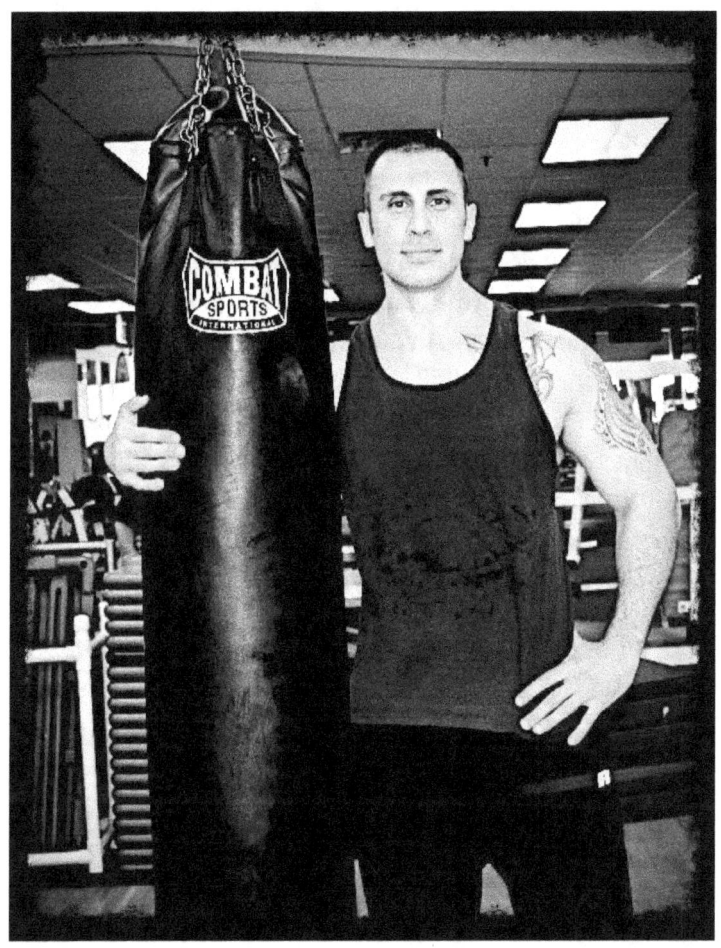

The power is within you; it always was and always will be. In most human beings, the expression of this internal power hardly manifests due to the false ego, which is the biggest killer of a person's physical, mental, and spiritual growth. This is because if your purpose is to impress other people, then your focus is on them and not on you. So you may get better, but their opinions and negative perceptions of you can crush your ego.

Also, as you further your rank or position, if your desire is to become invincible and transcend competition to be better than everyone else, then first recognize that there is no competition—there is only you, and you are part of a greater purpose.

There is nothing wrong with developing an intense burning desire to win. This desire is natural and essential for success. However, it can be a crushing blow to your ego when you learn that you may never be the best. It's okay. You don't have to be the best, you just have to win in life. Only those with this awareness can obtain the mental skills necessary to obtain power.

Always be a student with a keen thirst for more knowledge, more practice, and more progress—and have the willingness to pay whatever price is required to obtain your desire. A dedicated student learns the lessons, absorbs the contents, makes them their own, and applies them to action. This process is vital to this philosophy.

CHAPTER 2: NATURE AWAITS YOUR DIRECTION

Throughout history, many great authors have written about nature and her laws of **attraction** and **compensation** (which are one and the same), and how they relate to our choices and actions in life, for example:
- *The Art of War*, Sun Tzu[19]
- *The Book of Five Rings*, Miyamoto Musashi[20]
- *Nature, Compensation, and Power*, Ralph Waldo Emerson[21]
- *The Master Key System*, Charles F. Haanel[22]
- *How to Get What You Want*, Wallace D. Wattles[23]
- *How to Raise Your Own Salary*, Napoleon Hill[24]

After reading and practicing the philosophies in these books, I drew the conclusion that like a magnet, the golden rule of nature is: **whatever you give is what you get back.** I have seen firsthand evidence of this in my relationships with people, my wife, my health, my martial-arts training, and my business.

I interpreted the lessons from these great works to mean that **nature awaits your direction**, and this stems from your thoughts and actions. This knowledge is power and the secret to anything you could ever want. Energy can be endlessly channeled, harnessed, and transferred to other actions. Bear this in mind not only when you're applying intensity in your training, but in transferring energy into every living thing in existence.

In both my personal and business life, it has been my experience that when we continue giving for the benefit of others, we receive the same back. This will ultimately benefit us in the long run. Understanding this simple law of nature provides you with more power to give and receive. **We cannot give unless we have, and we cannot have unless we give**. This understanding enables you to give and receive simultaneously.

Every single individual is a joule immersed in a sea of infinite energy. Your soul is your consciousness, and when you consider that nature is awaiting direction from your soul, then you become conscious of your power. You can gain more clarity on nature through devoting more time to practicing meditation and feeling nature's energy within you. However, to become the creator of your destiny you need to make sense of your power, embrace it, master it, and fully express it. Once your soul directs the nature around you, the force delivers the results, which are the effects that harmonize with your original cause.

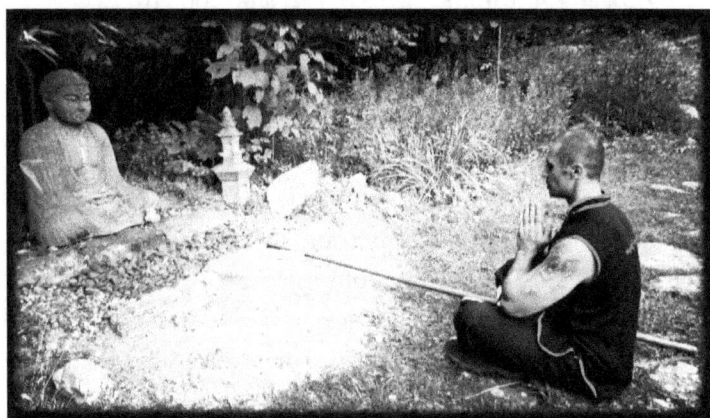

VISION QUEST

The world is a reflection of what we have within us. If you have harmony within, then love, respect, and abundance will surround you. If you have discord within, then fear, lack, and limitation will envelop you. The conditions and circumstances you often face in life are based on your **results**, because we mostly deal with or react to results. Most people hardly ever seek out the **cause** of their results.

At the beginning, it's critical for you to determine your purpose, because everyone is unique. People have different motivations. First, it's imperative to figure out what you want. You can do this through **meditation**—pursuing peace of mind through silence, entering the darkness, and finding the light.

1. Find a quiet room with subdued lighting.
2. Choose a comfortable chair to sit in, such as a recliner. (Comfort is important.)
3. Sit with your legs crossed, place your arms and hands in your lap and relax them, put a pillow behind you, and keep your back straight.
4. Sit still and try your best not to move. (You want to avoid distractions or any movements.)
5. Close your eyes.
6. Take three deep breaths, followed by slow and steady rhythmic breathing.
7. Allow your thoughts to wander at first, then when you feel ready to begin, focus on one particular thought. You may have to do this several times, especially at the beginning because your thoughts will often change.
8. Start with the why (**motive**) i.e. *I want a black belt, I want to be a mixed-martial-arts champion, I want to date that hot girl/guy at school/work, I want a brand-new Maserati sports car, I want two million dollars, etc.*

9. Continue your path with supporting thoughts of **how**:
   a) **Who**—People that can help you.
   b) **What**—The circumstances that you need to face in order to be, to do, or to have.
   c) **When**—How long will it take to achieve?
   d) **Where**—The places you need to visit to get it done.
10. Think thoroughly to know whether the object or endeavor is right for you. End with a fully-colored picture of your desire or purpose, *envision it in depth*, then open your eyes, smile, and <u>write it all down</u>.

There is nothing mystical or deceptive about meditation or breathing. The greatest leaders throughout history have been practitioners of meditation. Every single individual should use this great practice daily to develop relaxed breathing in stressful situations, and gain the desired results of their actions.

MEDITATIVE PURPOSE

There are different forms of meditation to amplify your energy, but to induce real power within, meditate with a clear, concise **mental picture** of the purpose, desire, or object you seek. Meditation must have an ultimate purpose, whether it's the creation of a plan, a vision of victory, healing the body, finding peace of mind, or connecting with your spirit.

As the mental picture becomes certain in your mind through **repetition** of meditative purpose, it consumes the subconscious mind. When you are active and have gained enough momentum, it crystallizes into physical reality through the laws of nature. But to receive, we must first give, and what we give is **effort** or **practice**.

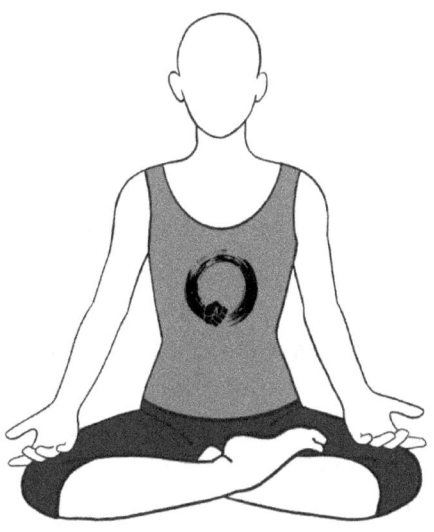

The following exercise is a powerful daily practice for anyone who wants to become one with the invincible power within them.

1. To begin, select a quiet room or location where you won't be disturbed.
2. Sit in the half-lotus position (as pictured), erect, with your eyes closed.
3. Keep your body still. The mind controls the body, and the body will never be still if you don't have control of your mind; it must be prepared to receive.
4. Start your meditation with several repetitions of inhaling deeply through the nose and breathing into your entire body.
5. Every time you inhale, push the breath down to the pit of your stomach using the corkscrew method detailed in chapter fourteen.

6. Follow this with a slow, smooth, and steady pace of respiration that fills your entire body.
7. Form a clear, concise mental picture of the purpose you seek.

Each symptom or circumstance we experience in life is an effect, and the cause becomes apparent to us during meditation. The potential to receive anything is within you, but your breathing must conquer all of the fear, stress, anxiety, and pain you feel. Do not let your fear, anxiety, or the trivialities of everyday life diminish your power. They can become a dark cloud that diminishes your internal sun. Conquer the darkness with your breathing, let the wind blow, and the dark cloud will drift away.

There may be moments in your life when excessively concentrated breathing is necessary to direct energy down into the pit of your abdomen. This scientific method of breathing is called **qigong**[25] ('chē-'gu'ŋg), detailed in chapter thirteen, and passed down through the ages to help people deal with life. It's not necessary, but it is conducive to withdrawing power from the world within you.

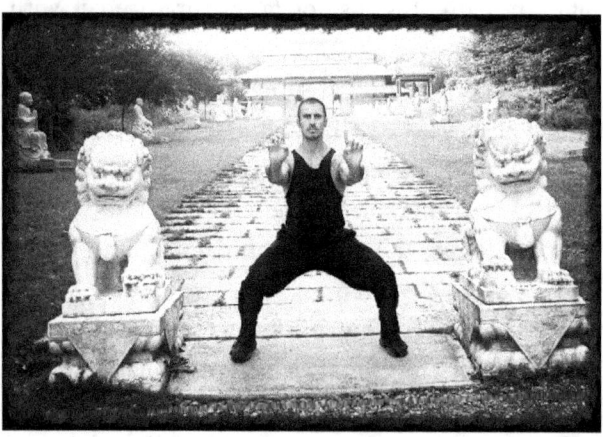

CHAPTER 3: WHO IS YOUR MASTER?

We each hold a strength within us that is ready to be unfolded. Our true potential needs to be developed, but sometimes it is beyond our capabilities. If our thoughts are constructive, we will seek a teacher to help us cultivate our power. If they are destructive, we continue to live a life of emptiness, misery, and discord.

To become a master of anything, first become an **apprentice**. Through years of apprenticeship, a student gains a wealth of knowledge. When this knowledge is put into practice, it increases the experiences that induce **wisdom**. Even when you think you are a master, you are still forever a student. You are <u>always learning</u>, especially when you start to teach.

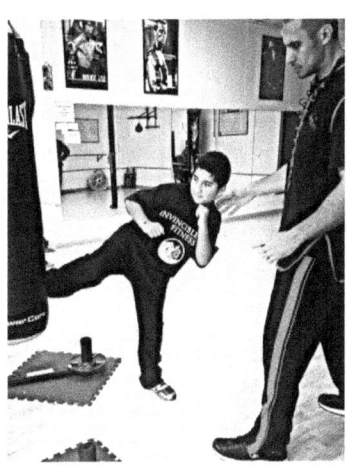

Your instructor must be able to stimulate your growth in the direction you wish to go. However, please understand that most practices are a <u>lifelong pursuit</u>. It takes time and patience for all material to soak in, so that your mind, body, and spirit can become one with it.

Every day, you must practice, and after every lesson, slowly digest and meditate upon it. Take your time and learn all you can before you take it to the next level. You will know when you're ready because:
1. Your teacher will tell you.
2. Your results will be positive, productive, and prosperous.
3. It will feel right to you.

For an apprentice, the master is the source of knowledge, and for the master, teaching the student is the primary purpose. The teacher-student bond is a beneficial relationship. The basis of the accord is **honor, loyalty,** and **respect** for each other.

This connection is the transfer of energy between two people, and it is one of the highest forms of energy transfer. It is based on the giving and receiving of energy. The teacher gives love, honor, wisdom, and attention to the student, and in return the student provides the teacher with love, loyalty, respect, and compliance.

The bond between them is a transmission of pure energy that helps to cultivate the power within each of them. Both parties gain as they feed off each other, and they simultaneously continue learning. This transforms into an endless cycle of learning to teach and teaching to learn.

WHO ARE YOU FOLLOWING?

A master is a specialist with the power to use their skills to teach others in a particular field or endeavor. They are the source of knowledge and the person responsible for helping you grow as a human being. A master is no different from the sun, meaning a source of security, truth, light, and love.

There are many different teachers in various fields. If we are passionate about different things, we may need more than one instructor. However, if you have more than one person teaching you *the same objective*, your mind will become cluttered, and you won't absorb any of the lessons. Likewise, **if you want too many things at one time, you'll never get any of them.** Confusion and clutter obstructs your learning, so stick to one source of knowledge and focus on one primary objective at a time.

Figure out your true purpose by knowing what you desire most, as we covered in previous chapters. Then, find out how to get what you want by talking to someone who already has it and is willing to show you how to get it for yourself.

However, don't just follow or listen to anyone—choose your teacher wisely. Some people teach when their knowledge is limited. Some "masters" are con artists who thrive on fraudulent or corrupt business practices. Some think they're masters when they're not. Some have lost their minds and their integrity, indulging in alcohol, drugs, violence, or sex with their students. Others have reached their success through deception and have developed a "God complex," and their followers have become cult-like in behavior.

The choice is ultimately yours of whom to follow. Try your best to follow reputable mentors, those who have genuinely helped others gain success and victory using proven methods. To find them, you have to research and discover someone proven in that field or endeavor using the following principles:

1. Watching them practice, teach, lecture, etc.
2. Talk to people who know them: friends, colleagues, students, former students, and acquaintances.

3. Read reviews about them from the internet, social media, journals, newspapers, magazines, and books.
4. Research them thoroughly to be sure they are whom they appear to be.

Find someone who is authentic and has the wisdom you seek. You can validate this by their reputation and characteristics. Hopefully, you will determine your master's character early enough in your tenure to see whether they can give you the proper tools for learning.

The majority of masters are salesmen and they need to be in order to market their services. We all, every one of us, sell ourselves every day. However, some people are professors of theory while others are instructors of action. If a master never tests their methods, then they may not work. If the methods don't work for the teacher, they won't work for the student.

However, *do not* blame your teacher if you can't achieve success in something you're learning or practicing, especially if other people prove that these methods work. If others have experienced success with this system—all things being equal—and you're having difficulties, then you are the cause.

If your master is authentic, with a proven lineage or track record, and you are unable to apply what you learn and transfer it into action, the likelihood is that it's you who is incompetent, not your master. The reality may be that you need to work harder.

Your goal is to better yourself on all levels, and in most cases, this takes time. If you are willing to change, adapt, and work hard, then you will develop the power and gain the success you seek.

A TREE NEEDS STRONG ROOTS TO WEATHER ANY STORM

It's essential that your master focuses on providing an environment to build the proper foundation within you. A **foundation** is everything for your development and is the basis for the type of human being (or in this case, martial artist) you become. The environment creates habits for you, and these patterns include how much respect and discipline you have for yourself, others, and the craft you're learning.

The potential to develop and withdraw your power depends on your ability to unfold it. Martial arts, for example, help to create and recreate the mind and body so it's ready to express the physical power needed at any moment.

Unfortunately, negative circumstances in your master's personal or business life can also have an impact on their behavior. If your master has built the proper foundation and you have competent peers and junior instructors, then I advise you to be patient with them. It's always best to give your coaches a fair chance by having patience and giving them time to cultivate you. Don't jump too early, because if you do, then you'll never get anywhere—that is a grasshopper's mentality.

However, if your master is yet to provide you with the proper foundation, direction, and tools, then you're off to a bad start. You will be undisciplined and everything you experience going forward will be chaotic. If your master isn't fully engaged in teaching you, you may have to get your education elsewhere.

KWOON-DOJO-DOJANG

The very first day you step into the classroom, your teacher provides you with the easel, canvas, paintbrush, paint, or whatever tools you need. However, **it is you who creates the artwork**. You are ultimately the artist, and you create who you are and what you want to become. It's best if you paint your picture based on your authentic self, because those who acquire power express themselves **honestly** to gain the full benefit of their power and to preserve it.

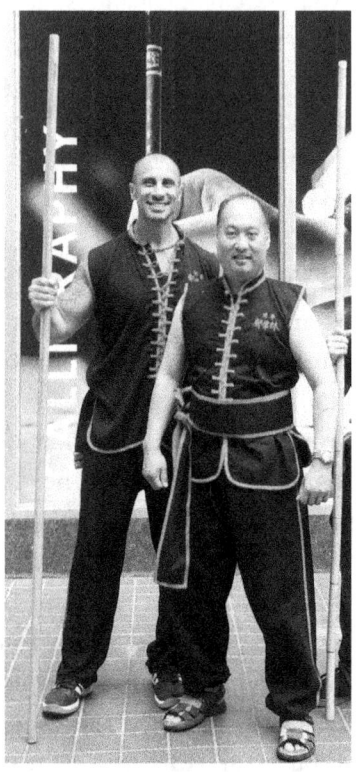

Your predominant mental attitude dictates the effort that you put into your practice, and this drives the results you get. Fortunately, we can rebuild ourselves regardless of our past efforts, achievements, or circumstances. A good teacher can remold the clay, enabling you to develop a successful career or life. For example, I was a classical mess when I first met my *Sifu*,[‡]

[‡] The term *Sifu* is Cantonese for "martial-arts teacher."

Bill Fong, but his guidance helped shape me into the martial artist I am today.

During your early stages of learning as a student, you are in the **recording years**. You retain everything perceivable by the five senses, file the perceptions, and store the data in your **subconscious mind**. The subconscious is responsible for your intuition and habits. Its operation includes everything we have observed or learned in our environment.

Let your teacher take you as far as you need to go with them, but never abandon them. **Loyalty** is honorable. Your teacher gave it to you, so it would be wise to give it back to them. (The act of giving and receiving is a natural law that you will learn throughout this book.) This relationship is one you can come back to at any time, and it can help you at any point in life.

Sometimes, you may find yourself in a situation or environment that doesn't feel right for you anymore. This might mean that you've picked the wrong teacher, school, or have outgrown their instruction. As a result, the methods may seem impractical, the lessons may not stimulate your mind, and your spiritual growth may feel stunted. Because of this, you may want to leave, and that is your choice. However, you can create bad blood if you don't make your intentions known to your teacher. If you tell them what's going on, they may be able to send you into a new situation that is a better fit without burning any bridges.

If your teacher is unpleasant but an excellent instructor, explains the lessons well, and makes you better, then it's fine to stick with them. As long as the experience helps you grow in the right direction. However, ensure that you don't take on the negative mannerisms or characteristics that make your teacher unpleasant. Never take your teacher's poor bedside manner to heart.

Some people can teach you how to fight or succeed—and they can be downright obnoxious about it. They don't have the mindset, time, or patience to wrap it up in a bow for you. If you can tolerate this, keep this in mind: one day you will be the master, and you can teach any way you like, but until then hang in there.

WHAT YOU GIVE IS WHAT YOU'LL GET BACK

In today's fast-paced society, most teachers have other careers, students, and affairs to deal with. Your teacher is no doubt very busy with their own life to deal with, be it work, bills, family, networking, or career growth. Their business or personal life can sometimes get in the way of teaching, and they can lose track of the moment. If this happens, <u>be patient</u> and allow it for as long as you can.

Your teacher's world doesn't revolve around you, but your world does revolve around them, especially since they are your source of knowledge. Technically, they may not need you, as they may have plenty of other students, a full-time job that pays their bills, or just teach for fun. However, remember that you need them to gain from their wisdom. <u>Never forget that your teacher doesn't owe you anything</u>.

It's vital to respect your master as you would with any elder, but that doesn't mean that you should let them take advantage of your good nature. You can be courteous, helpful, and respectful by listening to them and helping them out in any way possible—*without expecting anything in return.*

Your good deeds won't go unnoticed. Any help or support that you provide your teacher, even if not expressed, should be appreciated. Even if they're not appreciative at the time, one day, when you're no longer there to help them out and no one else has taken up the cause, they will appreciate your efforts. Sometimes people don't recognize what they have until it's gone.

It's crucial to not get lost in your tasks and duties. There will be no end to the distractions you face, but the key to your education is to be fully present and focused on the task at hand. Your classmates and teacher will know if you're not fully present. What's more, help others improve in every way you can by staying engaged. Therefore, engage yourself as much as you can, so that everyone can learn the lessons properly.

There may be times you may not agree with your teacher, or your ego might hurt due to **constructive criticism**. However, their challenge is forcing you to grow and raise your vibration to a higher state of consciousness. The lesson is given and received with the art of love, and passion for what you're learning.

Follow your teacher's instructions as long as they're within reason. If they force you to do something detrimental to someone else, then they have lost their way and it would be wise for you to move on. If your instructor holds you back because of selfishness or jealousy, or because you're a just a paycheck to them, then you have the wrong teacher.

The point of teaching is to **duplicate yourself**. Any negative occurrences mean that your master is unfit to be a teacher, and it would be best for you as a student to move on and find a new teacher.

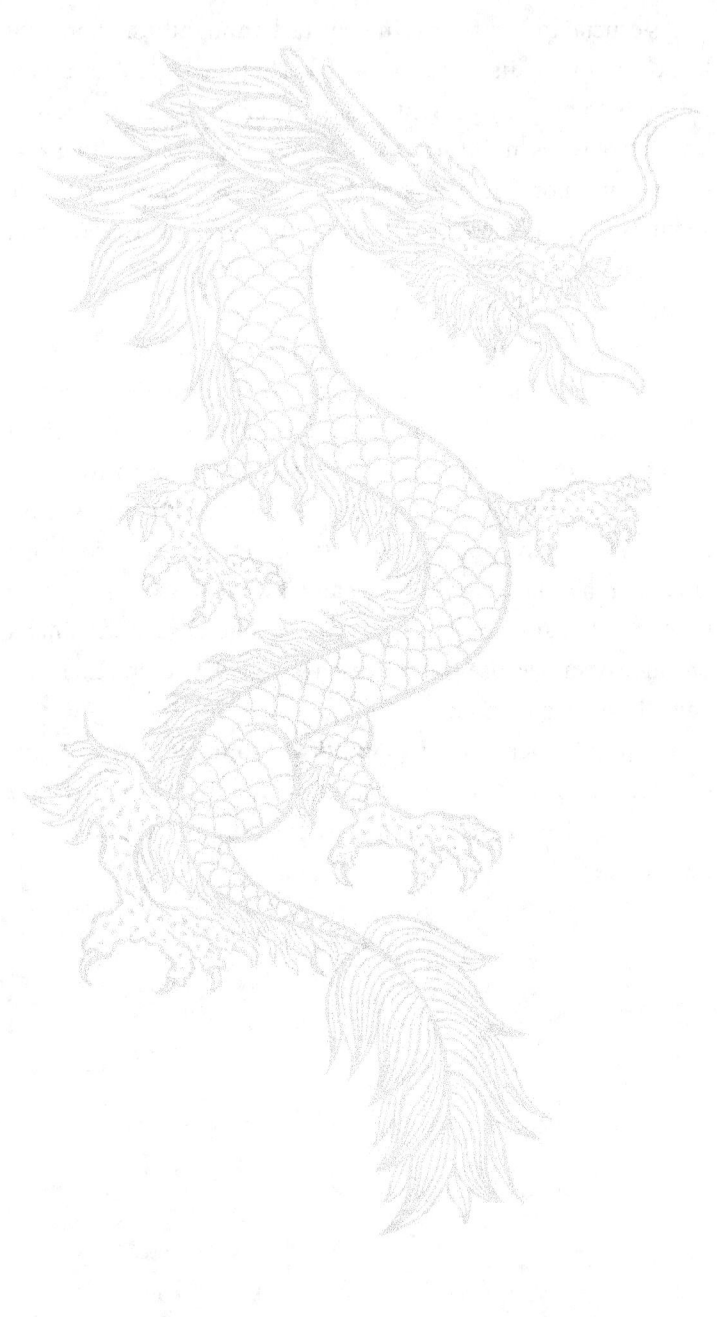

CHAPTER 4: EVERYONE WANTS TO BE BRUCE LEE

Bruce Lee took the world by storm with his words and actions. His movies were the ultimate inspiration. Since the 1970s, he has been seen as the alpha male of martial arts, and a symbol of strength and courage for people from all cultures.

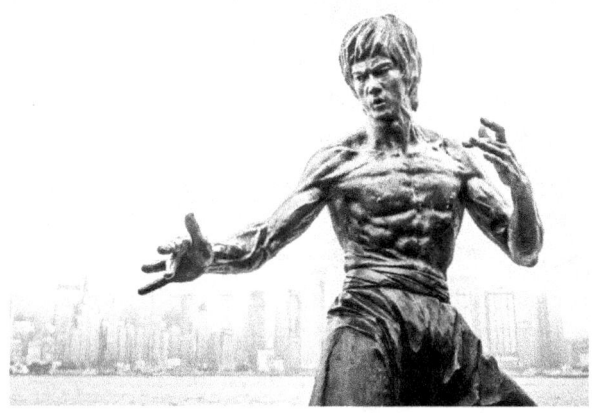

In his movies and books, he taught people many lessons that are still relevant today. Because of him, we know that to see better results, we need to develop ourselves **consistently**, and the changes may require us to go above and beyond our limitations. We can never change unless we are open and receptive to learning how—and this comes from within.

For this internal process to occur, start by answering the following questions:
1. How teachable are you?
2. How adaptable are you to change?
3. What are you willing to sacrifice to be successful in making the change?

Ever since Bruce Lee passed away, many people have unconsciously tried to become him by imitating him, fighting like him, taking his place in movies, or finding the "next big thing" similar to him in martial arts. They blindly follow trends without knowing why.

Instead, I believe that it's best if you stay true to your authenticity. **You can be yourself** because this will be enough if you let it.

MMA WORLD

The speed of today's world is swift. Patience is no longer a virtue because it ceases to exist with most people. This fast-paced society requires instant gratification thanks to the comfort of technology, which is the perfect distraction for the grasshopper mentality.

Most grasshoppers don't have the time, focus, discipline, patience, or depth to practice the mental and spiritual aspects of martial arts, let alone anything that requires total conscious presence. They are too worried about how others perceive them or how many "likes" they get on social media.

However, humility, tolerance and an open mind help you become receptive to understanding that one man's garbage is another man's treasure, and what may be right for you may not be right for someone else.

There are multitudes of martial-art practitioners who aren't training to get into the cage. They train for themselves and try to avoid trouble at all costs. All they want is to feel secure that if a confrontation arose, they would be ready and confident that they could protect themselves. There is nothing wrong with that. In fact, it's a core principle of martial arts.

In this new age, the concept of martial arts has changed to the point that enthusiasm in traditional styles is quickly dwindling, and the combination of **Brazilian jiu-jitsu**, **Thai kickboxing**, and **wrestling**, called mixed martial arts (MMA), has become dominant. These three arts are very direct and highly effective. Alone, each style is incomplete, but together, this trinity of combative methods has become a worldwide sport that became a phenomenon. Most martial artists are now forced to live in an MMA world.

There is a theory proposed by many outspoken advocates of MMA that these three styles are the most effective martial arts, and they could be correct for all I know. I love and respect them, especially jiu-jitsu, which I also practice. However, they have pushed the narrative further by saying that all traditional martial art styles are impractical and ultimately ineffective, which I feel is incorrect. Everyone has a right to their opinion, and sometimes these views are strategies to promote or market businesses.

Traditional martial art styles like karate and kung fu techniques do work. I see them used in almost every MMA match I watch, but most new-age MMA practitioners or fans of the sport don't know the source of their martial arts or the traditional techniques used (karate, judo, and jiu-jitsu are Japanese kung fu.)[26] To me, this ignorance is very sad.

Most MMA coaches and fighters repackage traditional techniques and pass them off as mixed martial arts. As a result, the traditional styles do not get the credit they deserve.

It's proven that traditional martial artists such as Georges St. Pierre, Anderson Silva, Lyoto Machida, Cung Le, Anthony Pettis, and Ronda Rousey have found success in the sport of MMA. Many others are making their way to the circuits.

The truth is that any practical martial art is useful and a mixed martial artist is not limited to just these three styles or the sport of MMA. However, it's becoming a common trend among the younger generation to pass over the traditional styles due to this narrative, when in reality, traditional styles like karate and kung fu would be great for them because they build a solid foundation and positive character traits.

Unfortunately, the younger generation tries to avoid suffering. They fail to realize that we must endure the trials *and* tribulations of victories *and* defeats, as these shape our character. These things enable us to build a solid foundation through discipline, honor, loyalty, and respect—one that doesn't coincide with instant gratification. **Everyone wants to be a winner, but true winners know what it's like to lose first.**

HOW TEACHABLE ARE YOU?

As we know, the majority of people follow trends, and most without knowing why. Every generation takes a new direction, similar to the fashion industry.

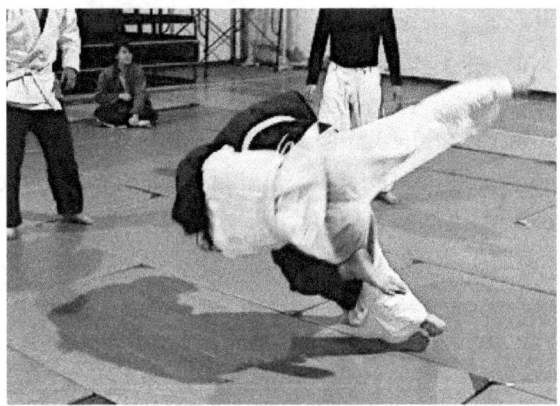

No matter the trend, **no single martial art reigns supreme over any other**. Anyone from any style can lose at any time. If you think otherwise, then that's your ego thinking for you. All martial arts are beneficial, as long as they help you to defend yourself realistically and are constructive for the mind and body, in the same way that musical instruments are valuable for growth. Some songs are sweeter than others, and some musicians may sound better than others, but music is an expression of the spirit, and the body's harmony comes directly from the soul.

The fighting applications of martial-art styles have to keep evolving as the theories of **timing**, **ranges**, and **angles of attack** change as people become more aware. As people develop, the moves need to as well. The evolving consciousness is forcing martial arts to become more practical, equipped with striking and a solid ground game. Overall, the combative perception is changing from a time when people were slower, smaller, or weaker, and didn't know how to fight.

Unfortunately, there are still martial arts today that teach theory without practicality, and they are failing to adapt to change. In some traditional styles, they don't teach grappling and actually exclude sparring from practice. In some jiu-jitsu schools, they neglect the aspect of striking, and in some MMA gyms, there is sparring but with limited defense or strategy.

In most traditional styles, there is a vast difference between physical, mental, and spiritual applications, and all three are mandatory to obtain power. However, most combat sports are limited to only *external* applications, so the balance of power shifts to only one aspect of training (physical).

On the contrary, kung fu and karate have so much depth, mainly as they include internal applications that the new-age mixed martial arts don't provide. Those who can learn, cultivate, and connect the physical, mental, and spiritual aspects may obtain balance and tremendous benefits in longevity (health and healing).

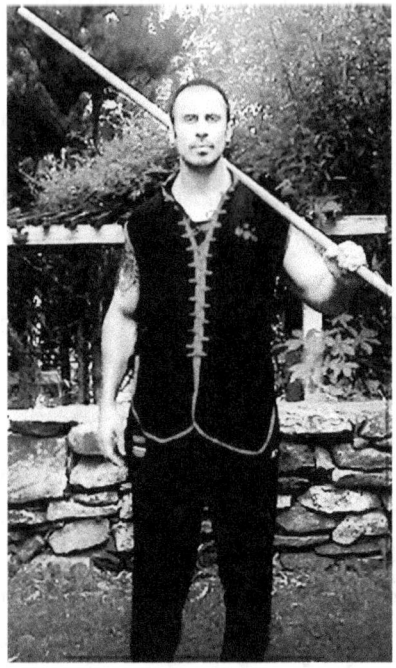

Combat sports are enforced by rules, yet some traditional martial arts aren't regulated for sport. Regardless, the efficient schools participate in full-contact competitions, and if you train in a traditional style, please don't deceive yourself into thinking you practice a fighting style when you will never do any sparring or test your skills on the mat, in the ring, or on the street.

Without testing, you are only considering a theory. When you have to use it for real and you fail miserably, you give the style a bad reputation. This is no longer tolerable. There needs to be a better balance of theory and practical applications if the traditional styles of martial arts want to survive into the next century.

Furthermore, if they don't adopt discipline, patience, philosophy, and the internal spiritual aspects of the traditional styles, new-age mixed martial arts will burn out when the threat of a new trend appears, practitioners get injured, or when a tyrannical government locks you down and declares that you cannot train anymore.

Ultimately, everyone has different motives, especially when it comes to learning martial arts, and the world would be boring if everyone were the same, so it's best to be tolerable to everyone's preferences. Every martial artist can benefit if they remain humble, tolerant, and open-minded. *So I ask, how teachable are you?*

HOW ADAPTABLE ARE YOU TO CHANGE?

The mind of today's human being has evolved and is stimulated differently from the days of old. Our thoughts are more dynamic and creative, and people are forced to think differently than before.

The human brain is intoxicated by digital and instant gratification, and as a result, the need for *more*, *bigger*, and *quicker* has taken precedence over time, discipline, and patience. Most new-age martial artists speak of discipline and patience, yet practice neither.

The subconscious mind provisions the brain and body. Our environment, our thoughts, and our actions are all predicated upon the generations before us. Our heredity or martial-arts lineage automatically forces an impression on our subconscious mind. Therefore, those who settle on a fixed system of ideas never expand, never evolve, and are limited in growth.

Humanity is continuously evolving; therefore, martial arts have to evolve as well. Today's martial artist needs both striking and grappling. Most techniques are valid; however, some might not be suitable for a particular person, environment, or situation.

Every technique has its time and place. They all need to adapt to their environment for measures of practicality like African and Filipino styles to the jungle; kung fu and karate to the street; boxing and kickboxing to the ring; and Brazilian jiu-jitsu, judo, and wrestling to the mat.

Thanks to the internet, there is no mystery in martial arts anymore. But the more we think we know, the less we learn. The wise men that continue to study end up realizing how much they *don't* know. Even a great master still has much to learn and can be beaten at any time.

Everyone is different, and differences in styles make good fights. When you know yourself first, then you can learn about your opponent. There are certain factors that make a style as effective as it can be, like the instructor who teaches it and the student who practices it. The more they both practice, the better they become. In essence, no system is perfect, nor is any system better than the practitioner practicing it.

Every day you train, you are further inspired, gain momentum, and understand the applications. You realize that your mind is creative, and all of your experiences shape your predominant mental attitude, which establishes your habits. These impressions start with the brain and the body follows with the expressions (actions).

You continually create and recreate yourself, and your world takes shape according to your mental demand. *Will you limit yourself to rigidity? Will you focus on silly, preconceived notions or fixed ideas about the potential of unfamiliar things?* The answers are self-evident.

KEYBOARD WARRIORS

In this new age, all of us have to be realistic. Technology reigns supreme, and the comforts that it brings have reshaped our way of life. So much so that we couldn't go back to the old days even if we wanted to. With this in mind, be cautious about how you approach the future.

We now have at our fingertips one of the most influential libraries of information known to man called the internet. When I was a kid, we didn't have the internet. We had to go to a library and search through hefty books called encyclopedias to get information. Now, we have access to Wikipedia and YouTube within a split second, and we can learn anything at our convenience.

The internet has become crucial to our way of life, especially in the Western world, and most people cannot live without it. This digital network has made the world so much smaller. People can talk to each other from the opposite ends of the earth and can communicate instantaneously at the click of a button.

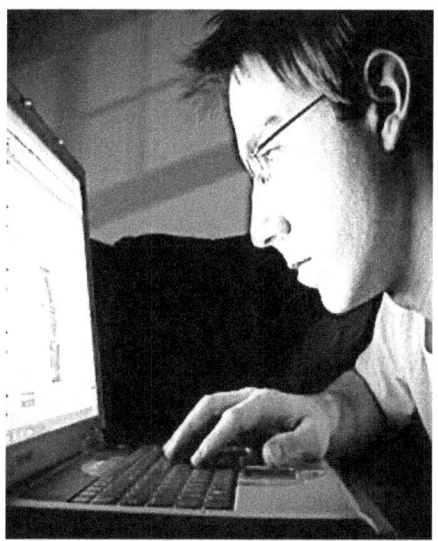

The digital connections between people on the internet have reshaped society in a way that makes us share our opinions, ideas, and theories more than facts. Through this method, "the man behind the curtain" can stay hidden and share their thoughts without consequence. This type of individual has become known as a "keyboard warrior."

The psychology of a keyboard warrior is rigid and mostly limited to silly, preconceived notions and fixed ideas. They believe they are experts at everything, are always right, and never wrong. Their narrative is that aside from the sport of MMA, none of the other martial arts are useful. This way of thinking is ignorant because you can say that about any martial art including MMA. There are successful and unsuccessful practitioners in every gym or dojo. There are also "badass" coaches or practitioners from other martial art styles you have never heard of who aren't looking to be in the spotlight.

In mixed martial arts, there are various competitors from different backgrounds who may have expertise in a specific style. Regardless, different styles make exciting matches. Now, not all fights go to the ground, and even the greatest grapplers can be knocked out or submitted. With so many different teaching styles and various interpretations of each method, any gym (*dojo*) can be more effective than another at any time. This change is apparent in all of the annual tournaments and mixed-martial-art competitions. Every year or two, there is a new champion.

It's difficult to get a bird's-eye view of the martial arts world from your cellphone or your computer, so it's best to try some of the other styles with an open mind before judging them, maybe even as an experiment. There is nothing wrong with dabbling in different martial arts. Masters have been sharing their techniques with other masters for a long time. It's called **networking**.

It's true that some martial-art styles are stuck in the past or perhaps not applied correctly, but there are a couple of primary factors in why a particular method doesn't work. These are always to do with the practitioner, their genetics, their comprehension of the technique, and the proper timing, angle, range, and scenario. No matter what, it's preposterous to limit a style's success to one single practitioner.

The real truth behind all martial arts is that <u>fighting is unpredictable</u>. Any martial art can be valuable if it can genuinely help you defend yourself or become a better human being. Unfortunately, lack of tolerance for allowing others to share and express themselves doesn't always go over very well. Regardless, stay authentic and be yourself. Try to remain open and receptive to furthering your education, and let your eagerness for knowledge be your purpose, not demeaning others. All martial arts are one.

The grasshopper who spends too much time bouncing from video to video never recognizes that each lesson comes full circle. Regardless of how much you know or think you understand, this must not mean that you practice any less, because training is the essence of all martial arts.

Ultimately, spend less time debating on social media and more time practicing. If you already know too much or feel that you have obtained mastery, then your teacup is full, and you are missing out on the infinite amount of tea in the world that can help you expand. Sadly, no more tea can fit in your cup.

Then decide whether you have the self-confidence to share your wisdom, even after it's apparent to all that your knowledge is limited. *So I ask, how adaptable are you to change?*

WHAT ARE YOU WILLING TO SACRIFICE?
Martial arts create structure and build a foundation for life.
A temple built on top of a foundation must be stable; otherwise, it won't stand for very long. There is a big, beautiful temple that awaits us. When we start to build it, we can make it look and feel however we want to, and it can be different from everyone

else's temple. Your creative imagination provides the material with which you build your temple, and this part of the mind connects to your subconscious.

To be strong, fit, healthy, and to think creatively, master the basics and never stop training in them. That logic goes for anything. The best advice I ever got was: keep things simple, especially when it comes to expressing yourself in combat. This concept was passed down from many different teachers and it's evident based on the legends of martial artists who perfected a limited number of moves by practicing them countless times.

> *"I do not fear the man who practiced ten thousand kicks once, I fear the man who practiced one kick ten thousand times."*
>
> — Bruce Lee [27]

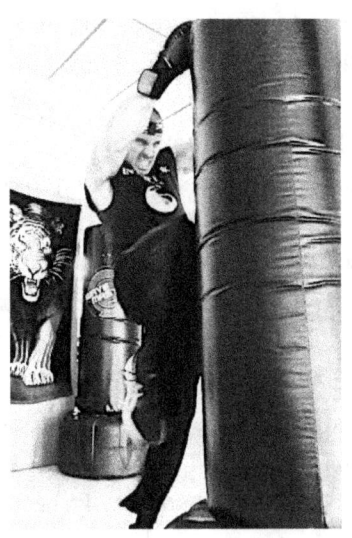

The martial arts are infinite and can take a lifetime to master. It's rare to find someone who can genuinely perfect any craft within a decade, but everyone is built differently. Those who grasp the basics early on in their training and continue them throughout their life have long and healthy careers. These practitioners can open the gates to obtain mastery.

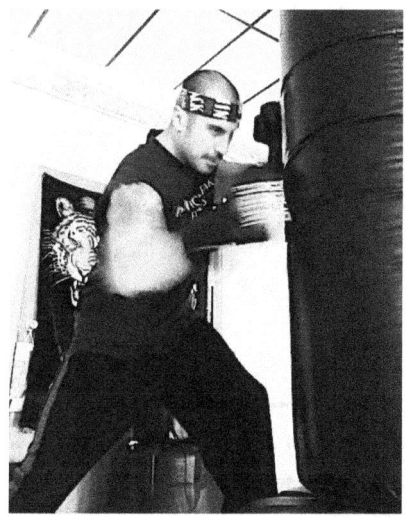

Practice is the only way to become good at anything in life. Training helps to develop the power, which unfolds from within you, and the art of practice cultivates this power. Practice each move or technique around ten thousand times (as a figure of speech) for it to be effective, to become a habit, and to maintain the correct understanding of the method. **Repetition is the key** to absorbing material in the subconscious mind. You have to practice these techniques over and over, just like anything in life. Don't just wait for class; it is crucial to practice on your own as well, and as often as possible.

Practice daily, digest, and meditate upon the techniques to grasp the accurate measure of them. This way, you will build on them and gain the creativity to expand on them. If you don't practice your craft this way, the methods become weak and the techniques won't work no matter what they are.

Try to be open and receptive to learning, continuously practicing and changing for the better. Practice for yourself, not for others, and choose wisely who you listen to or follow. The sum and substance of this is having your body express itself, by itself without thinking, in a way that has become second nature.

The x-factor in martial arts is that combat is unpredictable, and you don't know what the other individual is going to do. The majority of people are ruled heavily by their emotions instead of their intellect. This weakness is why you train for different scenarios—to prepare for any given situation.

No matter how good or bad you are, <u>being human means making mistakes</u>. We all make mistakes, but your power lies in bouncing back strong from those mistakes and limiting them each day you move forward. The process is ongoing, which creates progress and change for the better, and change is ultimately necessary for growth. *So I ask, what are you willing to sacrifice to be successful in your purpose?*

CHAPTER 5: THE WARRIOR SPIRIT

Martial arts are an infinite progression of expressing yourself. They are an effect created by a cause. The cause being man's purpose to become the best version of himself to attain, achieve, and succeed. He thinks, survives, evolves, and conquers.

The body requires **spirit**, and the spirit is the cause of power. *When you persist in your practice with no abandon, you will create motivation and acknowledge that there is no such thing as failure, and the accomplishment of your purpose awaits you.* But to adopt this philosophy into your life, first recognize its provenance.

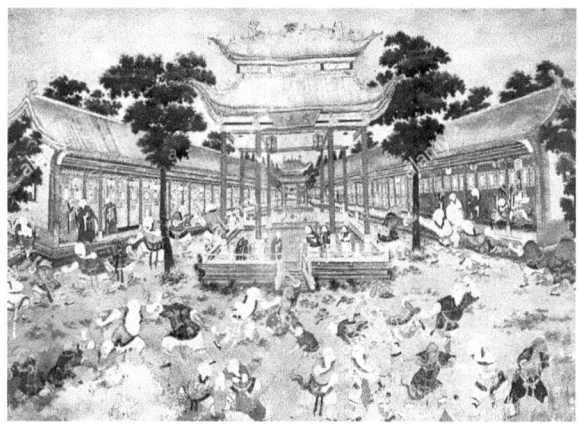

The origins of kung fu are mysterious. It emerged as prehistoric men sat around the cave fire, imitating the movements of animals. These techniques were passed down from generation to generation, including wrestling and grappling that was refined into kung fu. However, there was no system or structure to it. Eventually, the monks at the Southern Shaolin Temple perfected the martial arts into **five basic animal styles**[28] and practiced them diligently in isolation. As a result, they became the leading exponents of martial arts throughout China.

SHAOLIN FOREVER

The Southern Shaolin Monastery was the epitome of freedom from tyranny, but its annihilation was the primary objective of one man. The Southern Shaolin Temple became the number-one enemy of the emperor of China at the time. When you are the main enemy of a man with that much power, your hope for survival is fleeting.

Before its destruction, the temple became the residence of many rebels who despised the Qing government and plotted its overthrow. This rebellion was well-known throughout China and by the emperor. So, the emperor ordered the destruction of the temple and had it burned to oblivion. What's more, he had the nearby Buddhist temples in the region destroyed as well. Almost every shred of evidence was annihilated except for the knowledge safely stored in the minds of the monks who had escaped the destruction of their temple.

In defiance of the Qing government, the history and teachings of the Southern Shaolin Temple were recorded, memorized, and preserved by the monks who lived there. As the monks fled, they scattered throughout Southern China, where they were hunted and persecuted. Although their future looked bleak, they passed their knowledge on to the generations that followed.

In the rebellious years following the destruction of the temple, the monks organized anti-Qing occupations throughout the south. The teachings of the "southern fist" were practiced rigorously in secret and preserved as gospel to combat the Qing Army. One notorious group was the "Red Boat Opera Troupe," which disguised some of the monks as stage performers for the Cantonese Opera. Other monks moved to small villages and lived as farmers, tea merchants, and fisherman. They preserved the Shaolin teachings by passing their knowledge on to friends, family, and anyone interested in fighting against the Qing government.

Most people don't realize, or take for granted, the courage it took for these men to risk their lives to preserve the greatest gifts of life, love, and freedom. Those who possessed the warrior spirit kept fighting and continued to struggle in secrecy for as long as there was breath in them.

Unfortunately for humanity, the Southern Temple no longer exists; however, we still have the lessons, applications, philosophies, traditions, culture, and history that was passed down generation to generation from all of the southern fist styles.

It's a remarkable illustration of *willpower* that the Shaolin culture and traditions are still alive and practiced around the world over three centuries later. This lesson teaches us that staying connected with each other and openly communicating is crucial to preserve all martial arts. I advise you to take advantage of the full benefits of networking with others to get the most out of your training, not just as a practitioner of martial arts, but also as a human being.

Centuries later, almost every trace of the Southern Shaolin Temple is gone, but its remains are buried deep within the earth—and within the hearts and minds of people all over the world. In my heart, the Southern Shaolin Temple embodies truth, light, freedom, and love. It is the genuine "Number One Temple Under Heaven," and it will be the home of Shaolin kung fu forever!

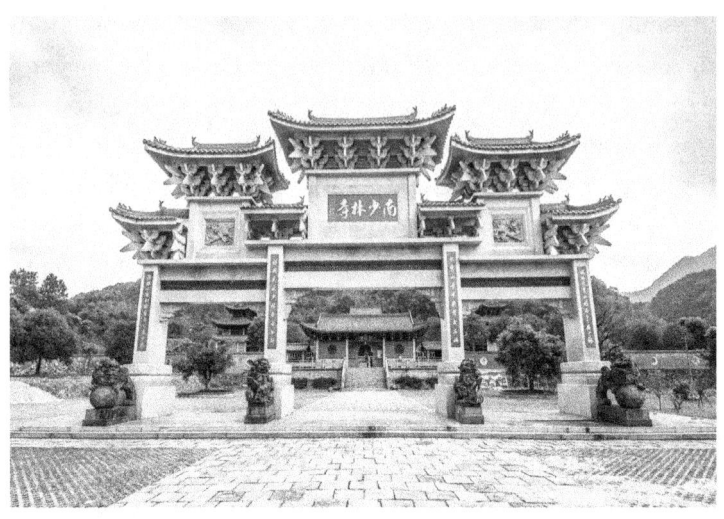

THE DISSEMINATION OF SHAOLIN KUNG FU

Today, there are hundreds of different kung fu styles in the world divided into two branches: **Northern and Southern Shaolin**. Whether north or south, most of the prominent Chinese martial arts trace their lineage back to Bodhidharma (Damo).

The Northern Shaolin Monastery is currently active and located in the Song Mountains in the Henan Province of China. The Southern Shaolin Monastery no longer exists. At one time, it stood in the Fukien Province, but it was destroyed by the Qing Army in the mid-1700s, leaving its history opaque.

Southern Shaolin kung fu has been divided under many different names, yet it remains available for everybody to learn. Unfortunately, the younger generations are losing enthusiasm in preserving these precious arts. Hopefully, as kung fu becomes better understood, less mystical, and more practical, there will be renewed interest in it—and current martial art enthusiasts will stop neglecting the traditional styles.

Kung fu offers many benefits, including **maintaining traditions, better health, self-defense, discipline, honor, integrity, and respect.** I often see kung fu techniques used in MMA competitions; however, the competitors, trainers, and audience are ignorant of their origins.

My teacher Bill Fong always said "Kung fu is not a sport; it's a way of life," and people need to understand and appreciate this fact. Kung fu needs to be remarketed and directed towards better lines. Thankfully, it's never too late to explore the depth of this ancient art and withdraw its true potential.

Most Chinese martial arts in the United States have been watered down and forced to adapt to the Western style of living, which hurt their effectiveness. The minds of Westerners are too focused on instant gratification, and with this comes a lack of patience, focus, and discipline. This destructive nature closes people's minds to the potential power dwelling within them, such as the capacity to overcome the persecution of a tyrannical dynasty.

Kung fu is the fighting style of a warrior, and its history proves that you must be a warrior to train its style. Its essence is a lifelong pursuit of practice, and because of this, a warrior's journey never ends.

Many people who grew up in the Western world developed an interest in the martial arts by watching Bruce Lee or the Shaw Brothers' films. Many of these people created a fantasy for themselves, where they grew up training in the martial arts and lived out their fantasies, but without putting in the work required. This work ethic was taught in the storylines, as well as the reality of combat.

Sadly, many practitioners fail to recognize the years of sacrifice needed behind all of the training to forge the spirit of a warrior. This weakening has slowly cost kung fu its reputation, but with new eyes and new awareness, and as the traditional martial arts evolve, it will hopefully come back to life stronger than ever.

You may have watched the old Shaw Brothers' movies, read the stories, and know the names and dates depicted. However, most people know very little of the real forces behind those names. You are familiar with the triumph, not the sacrifice.

You haven't yet learned from the great lessons so plainly taught in the shaolin monks' desire to keep their kung fu alive. Without kung fu, there would be no mixed martial arts, or whatever styles people practice today.

So, when referring to or training in traditional martial arts, please keep an open mind and tolerance for their teachings. Put in the effort and allow sufficient time to shape your practice. Give yourself the chance to evolve and build on the martial art skills you already possess.

MONASTERY LIFE

In order to truly understand what makes the Shaolin Warrior invincible, consider the impact that their environment played in their development.

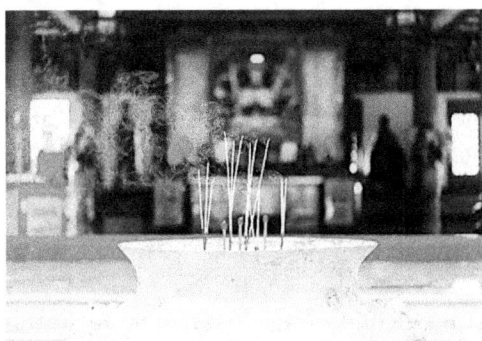

At the Shaolin Monastery, there were no clocks on the walls, only a bell to mark the hour, and sunrise and sunset to begin and end each day. The bell was the director of presence. Every morning, the bell would ring and the monks would begin their chores, which consisted of farming, construction, cooking, cleaning, laundry, and gathering necessities. All there was to life was hard work, studying Buddhist manuals, and the daily practices of kung fu and meditation.[29]

Their daily experiences teach us that if you desire to change the world, the change starts with you, and it begins with a simple task each day. Even the smallest job could lead to significant events that can change the future. Every duty leads to more functions, more abundance, and more life. In other words, <u>you have to work for everything, and the harder you work, the more you will achieve.</u>

The monk's work ethic instilled discipline deep in their subconscious minds, and that's how they were able to convert all of their energy into strength, speed, power, and focus. This type of energy transfer was needed to perform their kung fu properly.

Their way of life was a hardened reality: no television, internet, social media, video games, music, cellphones, fans, heaters, or air conditioners. They didn't even have indoor plumbing. Imagine no vacations and repeating the same day over and over again, the only exception new lessons to be learned. Imagine achieving peace of mind only after a hard day's labor. Life was tougher than you or I can possibly imagine.

These days, the word "warrior" is tossed around and has become trendy. I believe that most people have gotten softer over the years. They have become opinionated whiners, complainers that lack the discipline, attitude, willpower, and work ethic needed to survive in an environment like the Southern Shaolin Temple. However, their arrogance leads them to believe otherwise.

It's important to remember that the Southern Shaolin Temple wasn't a business or tourist attraction. There weren't any cash transactions, so you couldn't buy your way in or out of work, or use any sick days. You couldn't buy yourself a black belt because they didn't exist. It didn't matter who you were, who you knew, or where you came from.

The temple was home to a brotherhood. Every man was equal, and each of them had to do their part to contribute regardless of their physical or mental condition. There was more giving and less taking, less talking and more action. Subsequently, those who mastered their work recognized the influence that kung fu had in each movement and used it as a tool to perform their duties. The term "kung fu" was born when they discovered that the fighting techniques could apply to everything in life.

During their chores, whether it was shoveling dirt, lifting bags of rice, planting seeds, rolling a wheelbarrow, chopping vegetables, sweeping floors, collecting wood, or negotiating with local villagers, kung fu was at the forefront of each act. They understood and applied the philosophy in all facets of their daily routine. This realization wasn't limited to martial arts training or their work, it was their way of life.

The traits of kung fu are displayed when you breathe, walk, talk, work, fight, study, and how you treat others. It is the ultimate discipline. Learning this helped the monks bring everything into focus and apply it to their martial arts training. The desire to gain this wisdom created the **superior warrior**. Years of hard work and self-sacrifice were standard to those participating; it was a part of life. Their lives didn't revolve around the fast-paced digital age like today's society. There was no such thing as instant gratification or sitting at a desk full time, then going to practice for an hour. Time meant patience, patience took practice, and the training never ended.

The mentality of monastery life was unique, and the training was different from anything experienced today. Their conditioning methods were raw and hardcore, and helped them surpass their limitations. As a consequence, many of the monks suffered pain, injuries, paralysis, and even death, but this was needed to induce superior warrior behavior.

Today, plenty of martial arts practitioners don't want to get punched in the head, even while wearing headgear, which is counterproductive. You need to know what it's like to get hit in the face. It's the only way to prevent you from being stunned or shocked, and thinking you're better than you really are.

When the monks practiced, they trained to kill, even though the Buddhist tradition forbids taking a life. Since the temple was under a constant threat, the monks were only allowed to train that way to fight against evil and preserve peace. However, they were taught mercy and to seek forgiveness first, because every single soul is interconnected. When one soul is in trouble, all souls are in trouble because <u>all is one and one is all</u>.[30] This philosophy was taken seriously and carried out, whether it meant life or death.

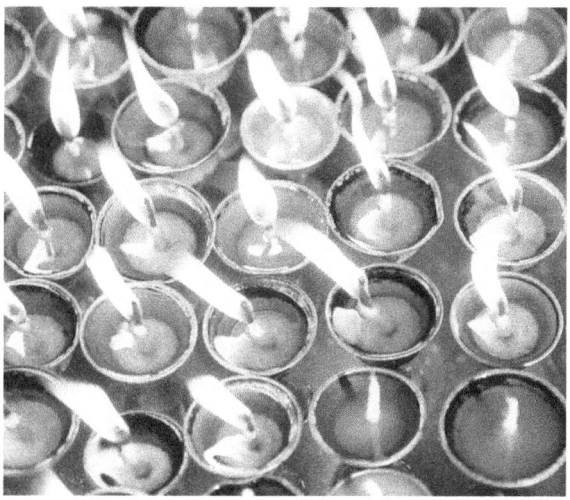

In those days, an honorable death was traditional, especially in battle. They accepted death as a part of life, which is the opposite for most people in today's world, who avoid confrontation at all costs, and search for ways to live forever.

The power of invincibility is the capability to die in peace, as the walls are on fire around you, and the burning of your flesh pervades the air. Meanwhile, you embrace the pain in accepting death, as you chant your way into oblivion. This immolation is how the head monks of the Southern Shaolin Temple died when the Qing Army burned down their temple. Their intensity is the embodiment of the true warrior spirit of Shaolin.

Death is what makes us human, and having no fear is what makes us warriors. When you finally come to this realization, you will have found the source of power that induces the warrior spirit within you.

GATE 1 KEY POINTS

1. You are the cause of your results.
2. Change in the world starts with you first.
3. Always stay open-minded and thirsty for more knowledge.
4. Find a teacher who has what you want and can help you learn how to get it.
5. Beware of false prophets.
6. The grasshopper is unable to think accurately and has a scattered consciousness. The warrior is focused on an objective; thinks with purpose, direction, and growth; and is willing to endure whatever it takes.
7. Be prepared to sacrifice everything for a change, which is growth.
8. Focus, practice, and repetition are essential for success.
9. Wellbeing starts with well doing. Service is power, the more you provide, the more power you will get back.
10. Pursue peace of mind through meditation. Seek the silence, enter the darkness, and find the light, as there you will find your purpose.

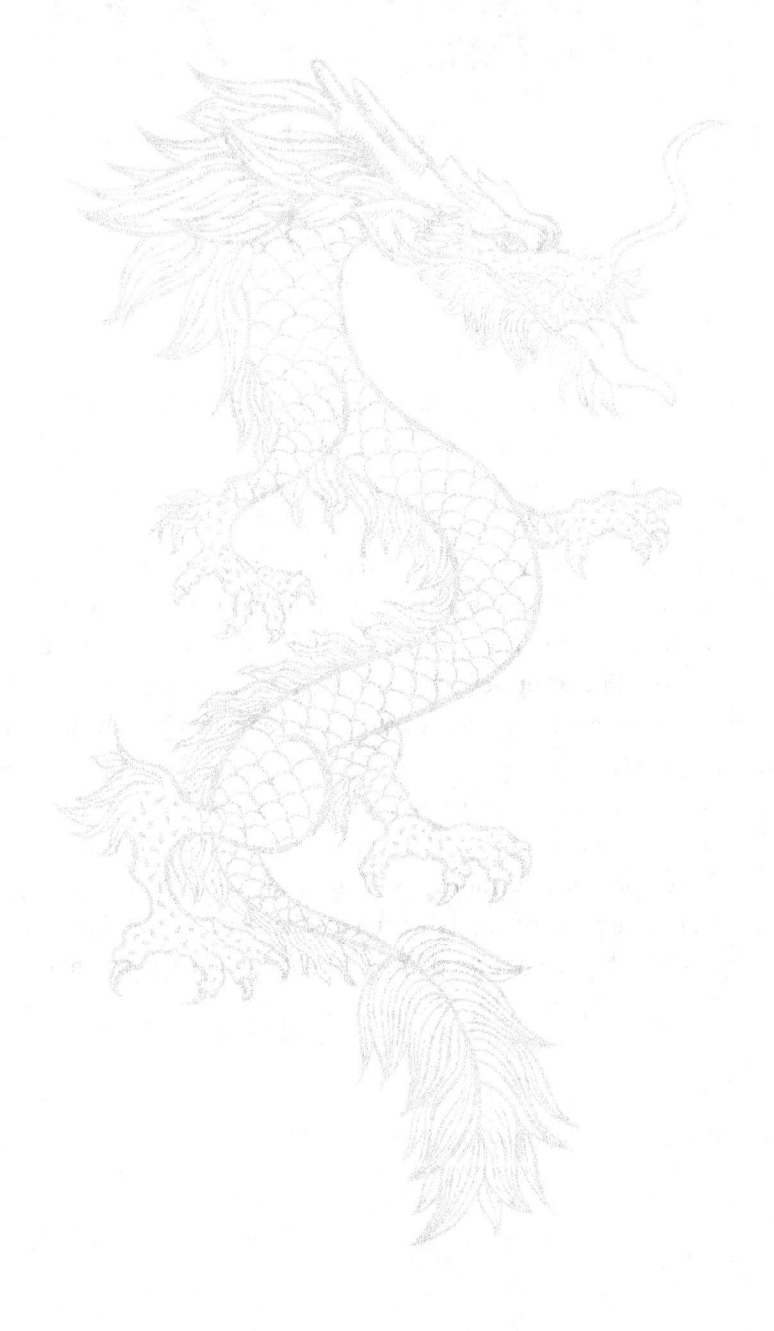

THE TIGER

When a fierce tiger descends a mountain and locks its eyes on you, it develops a certainty of purpose. It intends to tear you to shreds and make you its meal. There is no bargaining with it, no running away from it, and only one thing is for sure: it will not stop until it gets ahold of you. This form of persistence is how the tiger thinks and acts; therefore, you have to become a tiger if you want to succeed or survive.

The tiger is the first animal you learn in kung fu, because the big beast has no style or finesse, and so the lessons are straightforward. Although you may be young, strong, and virile, the tiger is naturally stubborn and rigid in its thinking and movements.

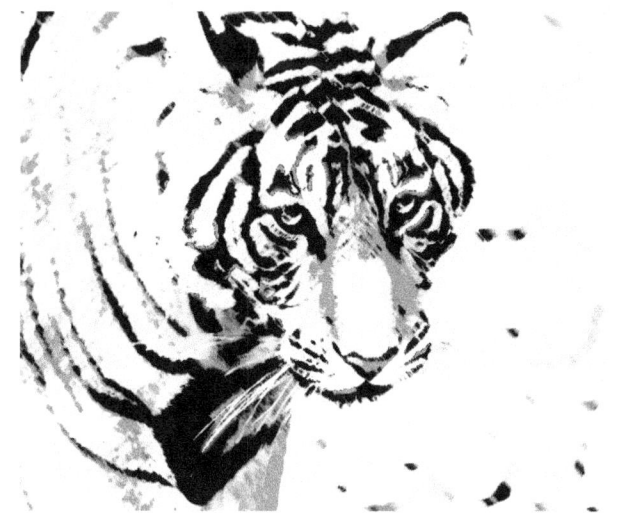

Luckily, the tiger is aggressive and persistent, and training in its techniques strengthens your ligaments and bones to endure pain. The foundational exercises increase your strength in the arms and legs. Strength comes from the ground up, and the tiger has a strong stance. It uses the terrain to gain momentum and develop powerful attacks. Furthermore, the tiger is direct, powerful, and explosive. When it's committed, it holds nothing back.

The tiger is like a fire, because in every kingdom in nature, there is a tremendous fear of fire. However, fire also provides light, heat, and security to the beholder. The fire element, which is synonymous with tiger energy, consumes everything around it as it builds momentum. When a fire is free and takes over, there is no stopping it. The same goes for a tiger, which is like a C4 explosive that leaves nothing but devastation in its wake. These concepts are beneficial to all young grasshoppers who are just starting their martial arts career.

Every single one of us has a tiger spirit within us, but it requires cultivation. The training of martial arts, weightlifting, and running brings out the tiger within you, which helps you overcome challenges. Think back through your life to past situations when you wished you were a little more aggressive, but instead were too shy, timid, patient, indecisive, or insecure, and didn't get what you desired. People who are more aggressive always have a better chance of achieving their desires, because they have a rare trait called **persistence**.

Everyone is different, and even if it's not power you seek but another treasure, your inner tiger will bring you what you need through a plan and persistent action. Now for the second gate....

GATE 2—THE FOUR FACTORS OF FITNESS

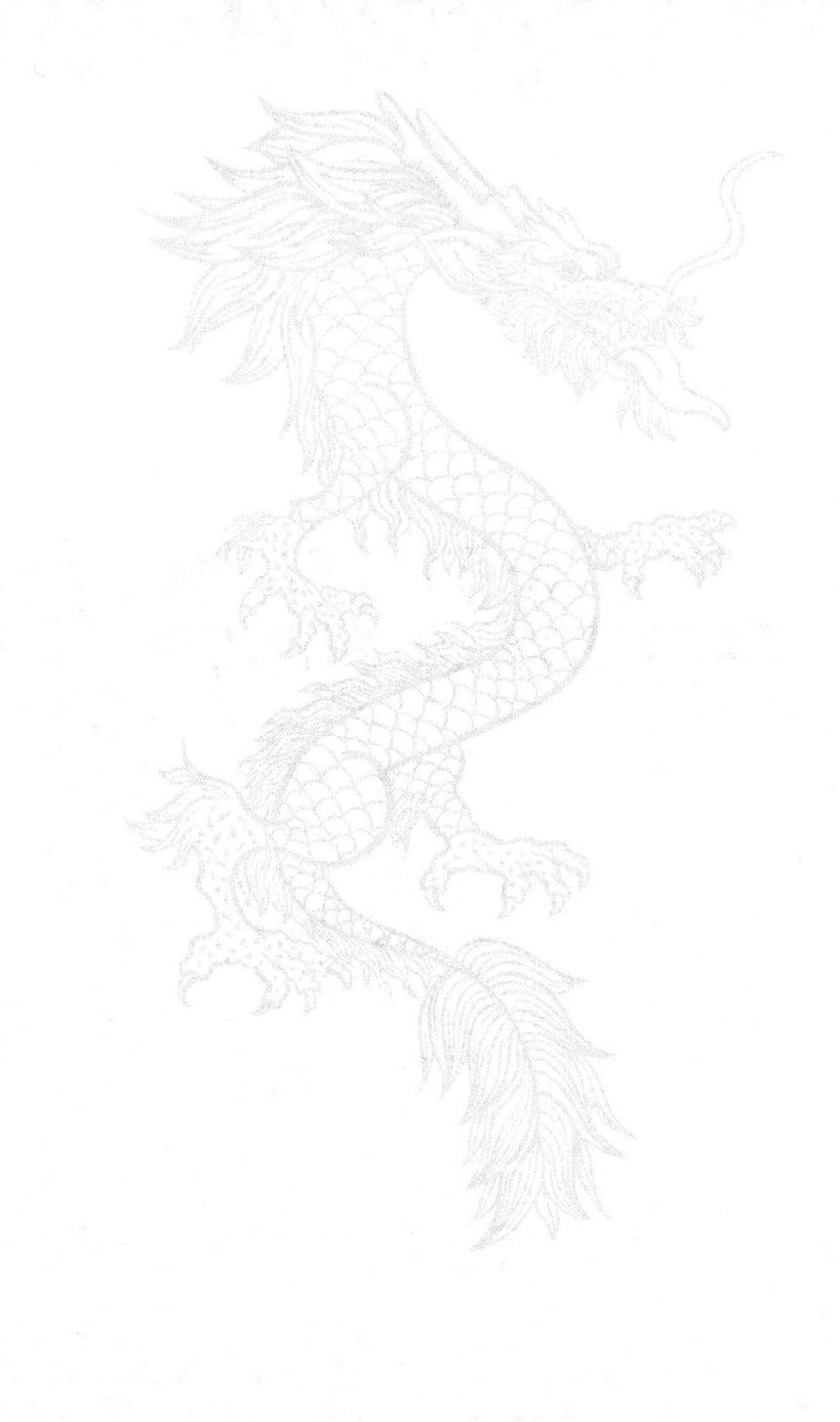

GATEWAY TO THE TEMPLE OF PERSISTENCE

Welcome to the second gate towards invincibility. This gate will give you a better understanding of how to develop **health-consciousness** for one of the most significant instruments ever created: the human body. Finely tune this instrument, because when properly managed, it may bring you excellent health, strength, and vitality.

To be in tune with your body, you must possess **good health and harmony within you**. Good health is a necessity for all, but particularly for those who seek power. Your desire for power will help you create *persistence*, which will help you acquire tremendous results.

Wise people state that all power comes from within, and for that reason, strength lies dormant within you. However, once it's developed, all of the productive forces and harmonious conditions that the body experiences are a direct result of it. Conversely, any tumultuous, unfavorable, or conflicting conditions are a result of weakness, which is the lack of strength within you as well.

It's difficult to obtain power if the body is always sick, in pain, or diseased. To correct your weaknesses, first seek out their cause, which dwells in your thoughts. In other words, a strong mind forges a strong body; a disciplined mind, a disciplined body.

There is power in our thoughts, so direct them towards disciplining the body, a process, which this gate details thoroughly. It's important to note that we must discourage and eliminate destructive thoughts, emotions, and habits, because they provide negative stimulation to the body.

The power within you cannot express itself if you are always busy with daily tasks and duties. It would be better if you found time to harness your power. Your power develops through exercise, and not just physical exercise but mental and spiritual exercise as well.

Practice each of these daily exercises without fail to induce the power desired:

1. The body requires physical activity and good nutrition.
2. The mind stays healthy with reading, rest, and meditation.
3. The spirit stays strong through prayer and positive affirmations.

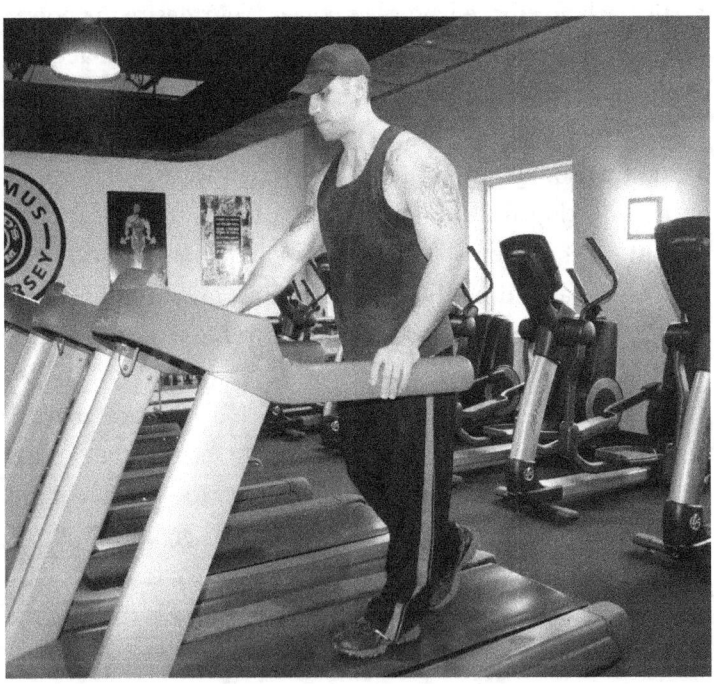

As a husband, father, and small-business owner, at times I find it difficult to keep up with my training due to my hectic schedule. There are some days when I have no time for training at all. These restrictions are common for many people who have demanding jobs, families to take care of, and other obligations. However, when I have free time, I take full advantage and focus on my body's need for physical exercise, even if I have to wake up earlier to get it done.

HEALTH-CONSCIOUSNESS

A significant portion of this book (not just this chapter) rests on the possession of **health-consciousness**. This is the mental awareness of possessing physical and psychological power, and it is part of power-consciousness (which you learned about in the introduction). It is threefold: physical, mental, and spiritual.

It's essential to note that mental health plays a significant role in obtaining physical strength. Therefore, to be fit, strong, and healthy, you must have health-consciousness. This awareness means that your mind is alert and obsessed with the idea of obtaining perfect health—that you can see externally and feel internally, so you can be at your best every day of your life.

Most people don't try to develop health-consciousness, so I have made it my mission in life to bring awareness to the types of discipline that develop all three components, which embody all of the characteristics to improve overall health and wellness.

In fact, many people throughout the world are unaware about the importance of health. When I speak of health, I don't just mean nutrition or becoming fit. I mean a trinity of physical, mental, and spiritual wellbeing. To be well, you must do well, and this process cannot be complete without benefiting everyone. The best wealth is health, as without good health, you almost certainly will not attain your full measure of power.

The process of developing our bodies to attain good health and power is based on our actions today, as this affects our results tomorrow. The development of our body is a persistent, gradual process that requires **patience**. Developing health-consciousness is not easy, otherwise everyone would look and feel perfect. So, we must not be harsh to those engulfed by lack and limitation. To inspire and motivate them, first start within, then proceed outwards. Always lead by example, not "do as I say."

Maintaining health-consciousness requires continuous effort. Day by day, as you persist you gain momentum and a better understanding. The plan you follow becomes a reality—your lifestyle. You feel no fatigue, display a positive mental attitude, and avoid injury and illness. You exhibit a highly energetic vitality, instead of pain, sickness, and anxiety.

Although it will take time, any student of this philosophy will attain physical and mental strength. You already have this power within you, it just needs to be cultivated. Ultimately, this takes patience to learn and assimilate, but it is attainable as a result of persistence.

To be fit, strong, and healthy means to find harmony within you. To be harmonious is to acquire energy and obtain power. To be powerful, you must be in tune with the vibration of power. Ask any sports coach or trainer and they will clearly state that a player's energy is only as useful as the mind it is attached to. This means that potential isn't enough to win championships.

Dynamic energy is powerful, and the higher the intensity, the greater the vibration. The strength and conditioning of your body will determine the overall expression of your energy. This form of expression may be the reason why Miyamoto Musashi and Bruce Lee overtrained. They were dynamos with the earnest hope of developing the perfect body to gain the power they desired.

> *"Study strategy over the years, and achieve the spirit of the warrior.*
>
> *Today is a victory over yourself; tomorrow is a victory over a lesser man."*
>
> — Miyamoto Musashi[31]

THE PURPOSE OF TRAINING

The goal of this phase is to prepare the body **internally** for the possession of good health and **externally** for the execution of power through strength, conditioning, flexibility, and nutrition. This process indicates that your focus is on feeling good in *every single moment*. It all starts with the mind, which then transfers to the body.

Please remember that <u>all power comes from within</u>, and this includes life, love, vitality, clarity, vision, and achievement. The internal world is where darkness collides with light, so pursue the darkness of meditation, and find the light within you. This is where you raise your awareness, though knowledge is useless unless it's directed towards a specific purpose. Knowledge becomes useful through **experience**. An experience may bring you wisdom, especially when you learn how to act and think in a certain way that makes it beneficial.

There are two types of exercise when it comes to the martial arts:

1. Training for health.
2. Training for combat.

Both methods include internal and external training. You will benefit tremendously from learning about how these two methods affect the different components, systems, and functionalities of the body, which help get the best results in your training. This is especially true with regard to the central nervous system, which most agree has more power than a supercomputer, and is the central operating system of the mind-body connection.

The central nervous system consists of the brain and spinal cord. Its purpose and operation includes: [32]

1. Gathering information throughout the body with regard to pain, injury, and disease such as the following: [33]
   - Trauma (injury and mood).
   - Infections (micro-organisms and viruses).
   - Degeneration of the brain and spinal cord.
   - Structural defects.
   - Tumors.
   - Auto-immune (attack of healthy cells).
   - Stroke (lack of oxygen to the brain).
2. Controls the activities of the body. [34]

The central nervous system also conducts itself with awareness, thought, memory, and reactionary behavior to perceptions from the outside world. This means it utilizes speech or bodily movements in correlation to the observations received from outside forces, people, and situations. It receives messages to the brain and after interpreting them, it sends instructions back to the body through the spinal cord to act or react accordingly.

The body is an impressive design, and the spirit within is the architect of it. Everything you have endured up until now and put your body through comes full circle. Over time, life has taken its toll on you and shaped you. This evolution is evident when you look in the mirror and see the image before you. Most people see the external clearly but neglect the internal entirely.

To change your results, seek the source. Every single pain, weakness, delight, or advantage we have ever experienced can be

traced back to these four factors, and all four are directly related to the mind-body connection:
1. STRENGTH
2. FLEXIBILITY
3. CONDITIONING
4. NUTRITION

All four factors are a series of ethical disciplines for living, not just training. Most importantly, they facilitate **persistence**. This characteristic is one of the overall keys to success in obtaining the physical power you seek. Therefore, a warrior must persist in his practices.

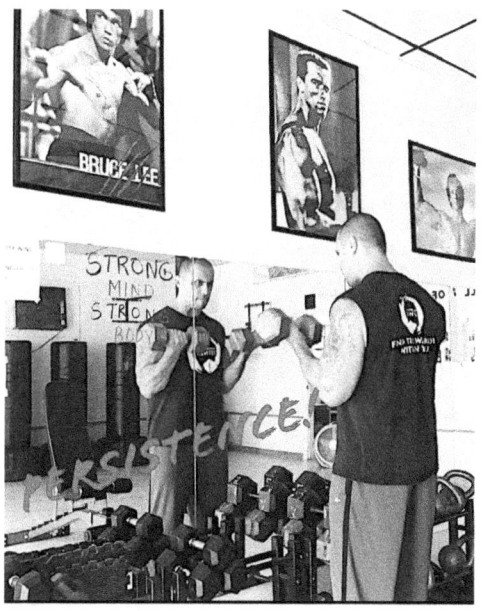

To me, persistence means consistency, and when it comes to practice, **repetition** is the key. You must become obsessed and prepare your body so it becomes acclimated to the intensity that improves your physical fitness and internal health. Furthermore, develop overall health-consciousness for the body to function correctly. Understand that your body needs to adapt to training through these four factors, and it will take time. Plant the seeds, leave them undisturbed, and give them time to grow.

The time has come for you to preserve your body and take your life back. Even if your physical body has started to wither, I believe there is still strength within you, because the force of the spirit is within you and your soul is one with it. In the following chapters, we will examine these four factors.

CHAPTER 6: STRENGTH

As we progress through this first phase of mastering the body, please understand that the component of strength is not just limited to the body, but importantly, it contributes to **a state of mind** and the brain functionality needed to obtain it. With persistence, a strong mind may provide a strong body.

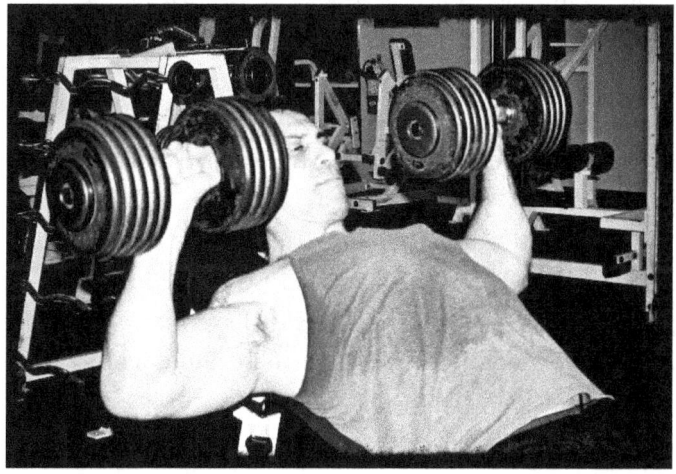

The characteristic of **persistence** is essential to your success in obtaining power. Strength, both physical and mental, helps to enhance this attribute. Therefore, it's essential to develop structural and functional strength in all areas of your life.

What does strength mean? **Strength is the ability to exert force**, which is the basis of power.

1. On the physical level, it's a demonstration of work ethic or action by way of bodily movement.
2. In the mental plane, it's a frame of mind that induces fortitude or a threshold for pain.
3. In the spiritual realm, it's inherent persistence, which is the seed of willpower.

It's vital to understand that your **tenacity** predicts your capacity for gaining strength. Therefore, strength is a predictor of your overall performance.

FIERCE TIGER DESCENDING THE MOUNTAIN

Muscular strength is an essential component of martial arts. Reliable and robust muscles are needed to deliver a technique with force. Strength training is required to maintain healthy bones, joint mobility, and metabolically-active muscle tissue. As a result, it's beneficial to do some form of strength training to develop the major muscle groups that support favorable joint health.

In the traditional martial arts world, there were old school philosophies of minimizing strength training because it was believed to make you slower, decrease flexibility, and increase injury risk. In today's MMA world, those philosophies are long gone. **The world has changed, and people are bigger, stronger, and faster.** This evolution is apparent, especially in the MMA world, where most athletes have reached peak conditioning.

Those who want to become skilled in any physical activity will benefit greatly from strength training programs. Overall, your skills will improve if you allow strength training to harmoniously blend with your martial arts. You merely have to find the balance between the two worlds, which many mixed martial artists have already accomplished.

Strength contributes naturally to your body's overall wellness and performance. Increasing your strength is quite simple: <u>make your muscles work against a higher resistance</u>. These actions will physically develop all of the muscle tissues in your body and help keep your skeletal structure in proper alignment to avoid back pain, as well as other discomfort in the joints.

A healthy posture is ideal for a martial artist to evoke power. Without it, there is no substance and no structure. Proper posture is a necessity in life, because it dictates how you feel in the present moment. Poor posture limits the radiation of your internal sun and can cause faulty execution in your techniques. This can lead to poor performance and affliction, which is why many people are always nursing an injury.

If you practice martial arts, you need to make your movements natural, swift, and convincing, and that's why strength training is beneficial. Through persistent practice, you can execute smooth, efficient techniques for both training and combat.

These days, you're not required to lift unreasonably heavy weights, and you can amend your exercise at any time. That's right—lifting heavy weights is *not* a requisite. Instead, you can increase the resistance moderately, even by just using body weight exercises called *calisthenics*.

You can develop strength significantly if you train intensely three to five times per week, for at least one hour per session. If a warrior lifts weights as little as three times weekly, this helps to increase muscle strength and size. Training any less is still useful, but the results are minimal.

GETTING LONG IN THE TOOTH

It's common for people to reduce their exercise as they age. At first, a warrior is limited in their ability to perform the same way as when they were younger. For men, muscle mass and testosterone begin to naturally decline over the age of thirty-five. This is why it's crucial to remain active and continue strength training, as it will reduce your trouble in performing simple movements when you get older, especially those required by everyday activities.

It's necessary to keep your motor nerves[§] actively connected to the muscle fibers as they age, especially in your twilight years. With deficient strength, it's easy to lose yourself (how you look and feel) and lose control of your body (your internal and external balance).

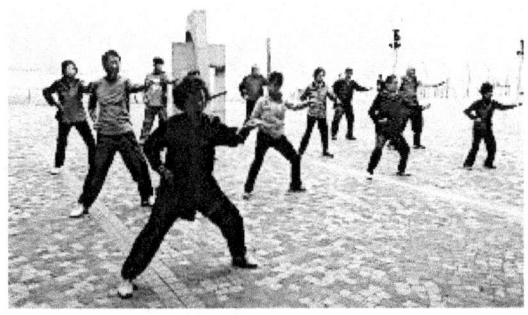

The premise of minimizing the loss of strength requires a full understanding that every muscle of the body has fast and slow **muscle fibers**. Every dynamic movement needs big, quick motor units[¶] while more deliberate actions utilize smaller and slower moving motor units.

As people age, the slower motor units in old muscle tissues start to dominate. According to a health study by the Department of Rehabilitation Sciences of the Hong Kong Polytechnic University in Hong Kong,[35] exercises like tai chi and qigong can be beneficial and improve health and wellbeing for older adults. Activities like

---

§ Motor Nerves: nerves that activate muscle fibers.
¶ Motor Unit: a functional unit of neural control of the muscular activity.

these keep the body fluid, and when combined with moderate strength training, they make dynamic movements less difficult.

Please remember that it's common for individuals to become inactive with age. Many people allow distractions and excuses to get in the way of exercise, but this type of mentality needs to vanish. The continuity of martial arts and strength training is essential for health and wellness. They allow your body to make movements more powerful and maintain muscle mass and healthy joints.

With a lack of exercise, it's easy to fall off track and let yourself go, which can lead to laziness, low energy, health issues, and injury. It is imperative to remain active and keep your body moving, especially as you get older.

HARD . . . CORE

Your core depends on strength, stability, and balance and is the driving force for the mechanics required to perform all techniques to their highest capacity. **Strengthening your core** is an integral part of martial arts training to create power behind your movements.

Martial artists need a strong core; otherwise, they won't correctly execute the techniques because their limb movements will be out of balance and their actions will lack the necessary force. Therefore, every movement, action, and expression of the body plays a vital role in developing strength. <u>Even breathing is vital</u>, as it enhances the core and delivers qi energy throughout the body and all of its organs, but in this case—specifically the kidneys, which are used to reprocess the energy for distribution.

Please understand that the core is not just limited to the stomach; it also consists of the lower back and pelvic region. These supporting components of your base are just as crucial for strengthening. However, if combined with weak abdominals, this will hurt your entire body due to lack of mobility, strength, posture, balance, and endurance. This is why the abdominal muscles are a great place to start when engineering a strong core. It's beneficial for everyone to possess a good set of abdominals. In order to improve their appearance and strength, first master nutrition, which I will detail shortly.

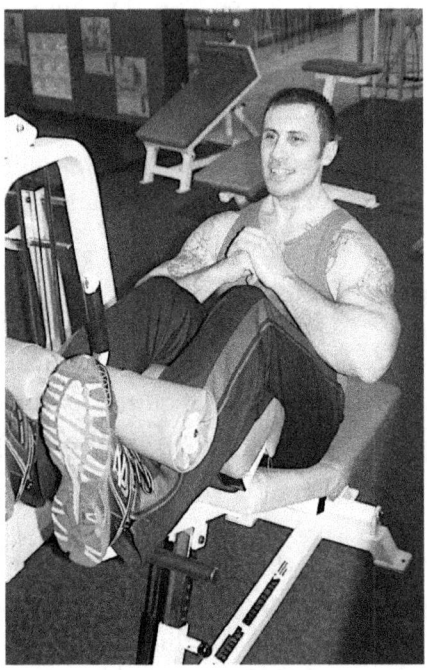

Although conditioned abdominal muscles look good, they must also be strong and able to take a hit. If you're a fighter, rigorous conditioning requires the discipline of taking hits, chops, or dropping a medicine ball on your stomach. Warriors hit hard, so your abdominal muscles must be solid as a rock.

Your overall training needs to consist of abdominal exercises, strength training, aerobics, and interval cardiovascular exercises.

It's also great for your core if you perform crunches** and leg raises†† three to five times per week.

In the old days of Shaolin, the monks would climb mountains and fetch water to bring back to the temple.[36] They had no choice but to use chores as a part of their training. Holding buckets of water was an isometric exercise that consisted of building strength in the body, but most importantly the core, as well as improving their cardiovascular systems.

As a result, it was common for monks to be well-developed in muscular size and strength. Their training regimens teach us that if we want to be at our best, we have to increase our strength.

In today's world, we have gyms with weightlifting equipment and machines. We no longer have to climb mountains or travel miles to fetch water. We also have a well-developed library of exercises on the internet to enhance our physical strength. Use this technology for constructive purposes, instead of letting it clutter your mind and drain your energy.

** A variety of different exercises totaling 250-500 crunches.
†† Three to four sets of 15-20 reps totaling 45-60 leg raises.

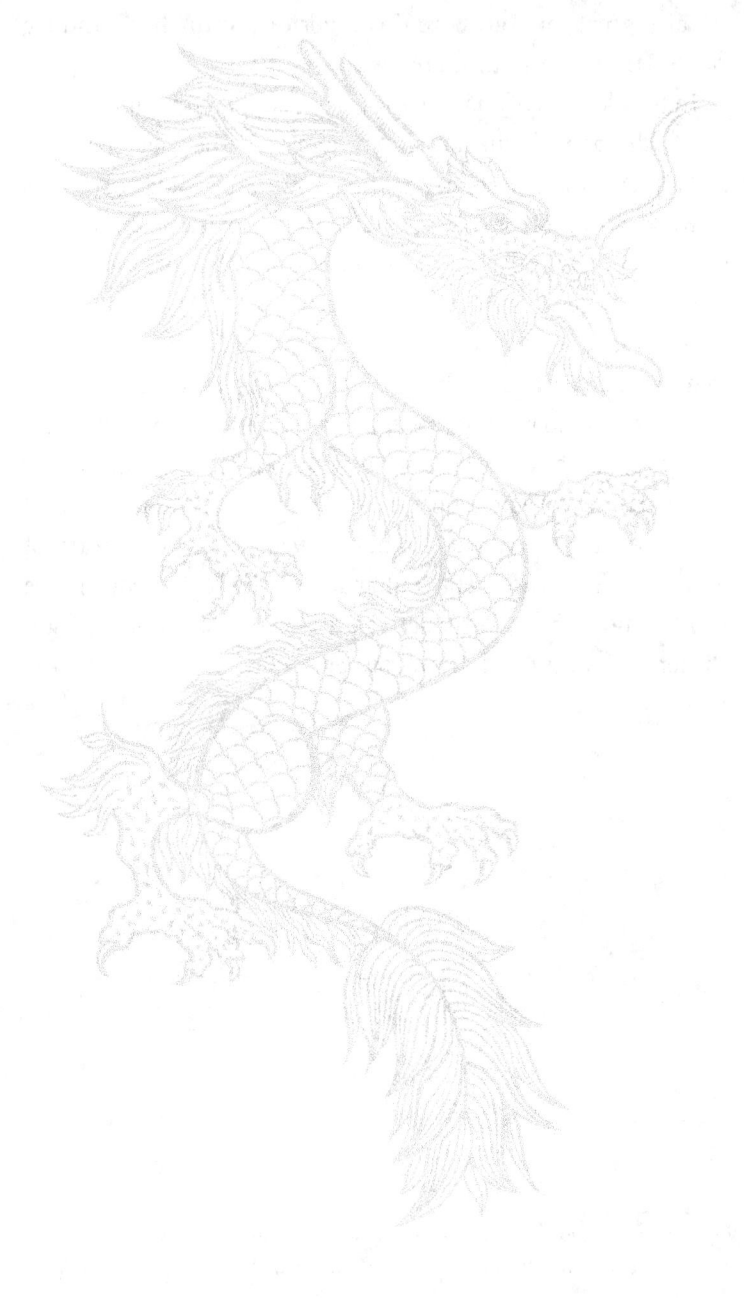

CHAPTER 7: FLEXIBILITY

When the mind is flexible, the body is sure to follow. But when it's not strengthened, the mind often plays tricks on itself to cope with the world. It's important not to get absorbed in silly preconceived notions, or rigid fixed ideas.

Eliminate the words "I can't" from the realm of your being. <u>Whatever one man can do, another can do as well.</u> There is nothing you can't do, because everything is possible until it is not, or you concede. The least you can do is try—try for the rest of your life if you have to. If you can think it, you can achieve it, as long as it's within reason.

The characteristic of flexibility gives an individual the ability to adapt to the ever-changing circumstances, conditions, and opposition they face, both mentally and physically. While we've been focusing on strengthening the body, flexibility is a harmonious trait for the mind as well. This form of harmony transmits itself into the body, enabling an individual to change or adapt to their environment. This allows you to stay flexible, versatile, and have an attractive personality, which transfers to your body.

In martial arts, movements are awkward and sometimes stressful to the body, and they may seem limited if you don't have sufficient flexibility. This dictates the capacity that an individual has to move a joint through its full range of motion, which is an important attribute for improving overall health and performance.

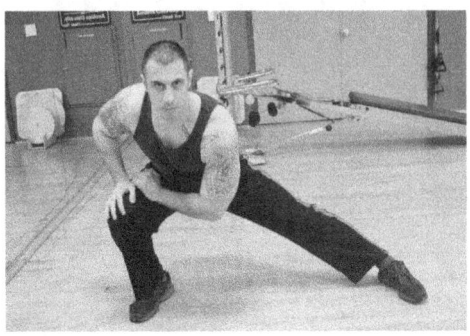

Flexibility is essential for standard joint functionality and provides smooth movements with an economy of motion. The majority of our aches and pains reside in the joints due to blockages or tissues that obstruct our range of motion. Flexibility helps to remove these blockages and recuperate the body, leading to good health and optimal performance.

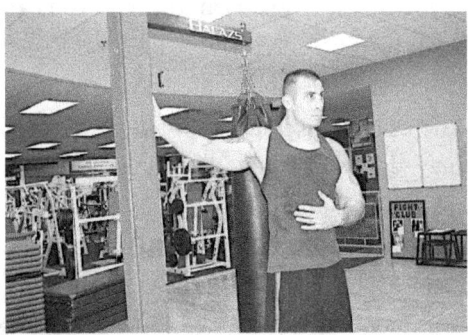

Flexibility is necessary to maintain the health of all your major joints. Furthermore, it helps to keep your bones and muscles in proper alignment, which assists with **injury prevention**. Strengthening the knees, shoulders, wrists, and ankles is crucial to prevent unnecessary stress and helps support muscle groups and soft tissues. This will assist your body in staying pain-free.

Remember, your goal is to feel good in every moment, so a pain-free body makes for a positive and healthy frame of mind. People lose elasticity if they don't stretch consistently or move their joints regularly through normal ranges of motion. For this reason, it's necessary to keep active. Once you lose flexibility, it's more challenging to restore. Subsequently, it's crucial to stay consistent with stretching and exercise to maintain your flexibility.

HAND BENDS A CINNAMON TREE

The muscles have an elasticity to them that is similar to a rubber band, and muscle tissue is one of the essential keys to developing flexibility. Muscle tissue is divided into two forms:[37]

1. **Elastin fibers** which are elastic and flexible, allowing the muscles to stretch.
2. **Collagen fibers** which provide structure, support, and help to stop the tissue from extending too far.

It's beneficial to stretch before *and* after training. Slow extension improves your flexibility and explosiveness in all movements. However, there needs to be a balance between these muscle fibers, because even overstretching can trigger severe injury.

Youthful practitioners are likely to avoid the practice of stretching and elude consequence, but it's essential to know that as the body matures, it becomes more susceptible to injury. This fact should be a high priority for everyone, especially martial artists, because flexibility plays a significant role in releasing explosive power.

The muscle fibers that create explosive movements must not be limited, yet they must grow longer in a safe manner that promotes the economy of motion. These dynamics are crucial for the maximum benefit of every action. Think of a snake and how it coils before it strikes its prey.

Expansion and contraction is key in combat, especially when reading opponents' movements and learning their timing so you may counter accordingly.

GOLDEN LEOPARD STRETCHES THE SPINE

Aerobic and cardiovascular exercises are not only favorable for improving stamina, but also useful for strengthening the leg muscles and improving overall mobility. Activities such as walking, jogging, jumping rope, slow katas (forms), yoga (vinyasa flow), qigong, and tai chi are great for a warm-up before your actual training commences. Perform movements that allow your joints and skeletal system supporting structures to loosen quickly and effortlessly.

Once the body is warm, the muscles are ready for stretching. Our joints connect our bones, and performing natural movements helps to loosen them up for exercise. This increases our support in all actions and allows our muscles to function more efficiently, which helps to prevent injuries.

Basic stretching is essential, but the martial arts have a variety of specific stretches that improve flexibility for maximum performance. Since Bodhidharma was a yoga practitioner, a lot of the poses built into kung fu derive from yoga, and they not only develop flexibility, but increase blood circulation as well.

There are three types of basic stretching:

1. **Static**: Slow and gradual poses that take between ten and thirty seconds. (The isometric poses in stretching sessions practiced by yogis, martial artists, gymnasts, and dancers usually go on for longer periods.)
2. **Ballistic:** Dynamic movements where the muscles are stretched abruptly in a bouncing movement.
3. **Passive:** Partnered stretching.

Static and ballistic are the two most commonly used stretches. Static stretching is the safest and most effective method. These stretches increase joint mobility without intensifying sensitivity to the stretch receptors.

In ballistic stretching, if the response from the stretch receptors is too robust, it can cause injury, so the bouncing movements during stretching aren't ideal. Passive stretching is valuable and used by experienced practitioners who have excellent communication skills and thoroughly understand the methods. At the Shaolin Monastery, the monks would sometimes utilize passive stretches to help a beginner perform splits or other exotic stretches. However, those who receive passive stretches lack movement control and are at increased risk of injury.

There is a link between strength and flexibility—and if you only want to gain strength, then a minimal amount of flexibility is required. However, if your flexibility is very poor, then your quest for power won't be attained as easily.

At one time, there was a philosophy that lifting weights made an individual too muscular or too slow to perform some of the necessary movements in martial arts. However, in my studies, I found that Bruce Lee[38] and James Yimm Lee[39] were two of the few outspoken advocates who openly promoted weightlifting as a form of compensatory training to martial arts. Furthermore, as I delved deeper into the history of Southern Shaolin kung fu, I discovered that weightlifting exercises were an elemental factor in their training too.

Many bodybuilders and weightlifters have large, bulky muscles because they sacrifice flexibility for muscle size and strength. On the other hand, many of the Shaolin monks were able to possess both attributes in their martial arts training, which allowed them to be elite fighters throughout China.

In today's world, athletes, boxers, kickboxers, and mixed martial artists have found a good balance between the two components and display them in sport or combat. It is possible to have high strength and sufficient flexibility simultaneously; however, persistently work at it through the following fundamentals:

1. Practice warm-up exercises such as walking, jogging, calisthenics, or jump rope before attempting a stretching routine.
2. Practice stretching daily to gradually develop your flexibility.
3. Practice static stretching exercises by holding each pose for ten-thirty seconds and try not to bounce when stretching to avoid risk of injury. (Yoga, qigong, martial arts, gymnastics, and dancing may have varying methods of rocking or eccentric movements to settle in the stretching pose—regardless, use caution.)
4. Stay relaxed and breathe while stretching to prevent pain.
5. Practice symmetry by stretching all of the major joints and limbs, and on both sides of the body.

CHAPTER 8: CONDITIONING

In life, it's essential to create realistic goals for yourself, whether it's for attainment, achievement, or success. Everyone's goals are different; however, in your development, know your edge and never pretend to be more than you are.

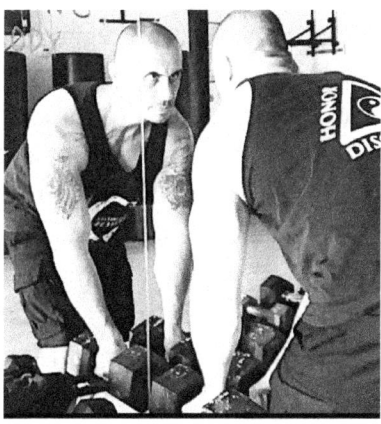

It's okay to admit your fears, know your limitations, and still pursue your capacity for growth and development. No matter what, face your fears openly and willingly in your quest for power because any form of ego or deceit will come back to haunt you through negative karma.

Power is success, security, and freedom to live without fear. If training for power is your cause, then both the novice and expert seek the same results. Both subject themselves to extreme stress so the mind increases functionality in the brain to express action, and the body responds and adapts by improving its performance. This process takes the psychological conditioning of willpower and persistence.

It's beneficial to have a stable twelve-week conditioning program, but it requires knowledge of the effects that each exercise has on the body. A practitioner improves when their body acclimates to the specific stress needed to endure their purpose. For example, training for a sport and preparing for survival are two different things. The preparations for each depend explicitly on the environment or rules in place, and how much time you have to prepare.

In a sports competition, there are rules and guidelines to follow, thus training is periodized and regimented for longevity. However, on the street there are no rules, so combat is unpredictable and practice is for survival. Preparation for either one has limited transferability to the other because they are based on two different premises: one is for sport (competition and entertainment) and the other for survival (self-preservation).

It's difficult to gauge your progress in training without the validity of competition. For example, if you are continually practicing theory without sparring, there will be very little transfer of effectiveness because everything is hypothetical. If you are in a system that helps to distinguish fact from theory, and you're able to utilize the techniques for survival on the street or performance in sport, then this system is effective for whatever environment you inhabit.

If you practice consistently and aren't able to transfer the techniques to the environment, then either the system is wrong for you, or you are unsuitable for the system. Either way, your results will be interpreted in the aftermath, and you decide whether to accept failure and continue to practice or seek other methods more suitable to your abilities.

THE COMPONENTS OF POWER

The critical components of conditioning are: explosiveness, speed, strength, endurance, agility, flexibility, bone density, and aerobic capacity. All of them are crucial to your overall performance.[40] However, everyone is built differently and learns distinctively. Therefore, genetics can be a huge factor in limiting your interpretation, skill, and execution.

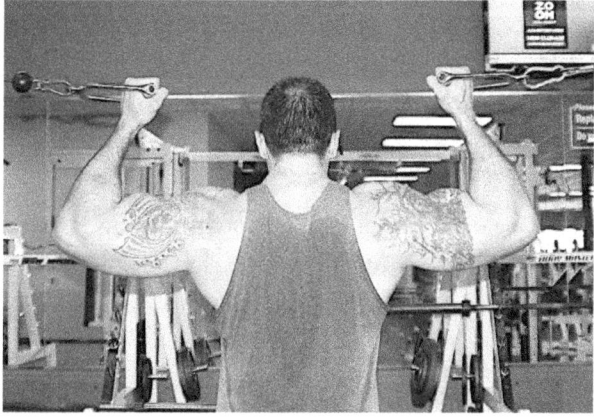

Some people are physically bigger and stronger, while others are smaller and faster. Some need time to practice and digest the material and others just "get it" right away, so the progression to adaptation from training may take longer for some than others.

The legends, past and present, were born with a capacity to produce significant power with their techniques. Their genetics helped to create "geniuses" in the martial arts world. These elite warriors started their training at a much higher level than everyone else. Unfortunately, average people can't expect to duplicate their physical abilities no matter how hard they train. However, *anyone* can improve their skill in strength, agility, and speed if they develop power. Either way, power development takes continuous conditioning, both physically and mentally.

TRAINING VARIATIONS

According to the first principle of the seven "granddaddy" laws of the International Sports Sciences Association (ISSA),[41] **the principle of individual differences,** we all have different genetics and not everyone adapts to or responds to training in the same manner. The rate and magnitude of change, growth, and development varies with each individual. It's important to experiment with different training methods for two reasons:

1. To create realistic goals.
2. To avoid the frustration of not seeing any change in your body or performance.

We all have different needs, and you have to find what works best for you. In my younger days, I received various training tips from different mentors. Following the Joe Weider System of weight training (which has been in place for over fifty years), I found some of the principles beneficial in improving my training:[42]

1. **Double or triple-split training:** Breaking your workout down into two or three shorter, more intense training sessions per day.
2. **Muscle confusion principle:** Muscles adapt to specific types of stress over time and eventually plateau, so you constantly vary exercises, sets, repetitions, and weight to avoid adaptation.[43]

Some of these principles were very common among my peers in bodybuilding. In addition, I follow the training philosophies of Southern Shaolin, Musashi, and Bruce Lee, which are all similar. I have found it beneficial to change my routines, the activities I choose, and the time of day I train—even training when I am tired.

An old, stale routine can have adverse effects that limit your growth and ability to execute the moves. All of these forms of training may improve your overall athleticism, so please don't get stuck on old habits or stale routines. We have to climb higher and higher, especially in today's competitive world. Learning how to maximize the performance of your muscles and supporting joints can enhance your motion. What's more, muscles react differently to particular training programs.

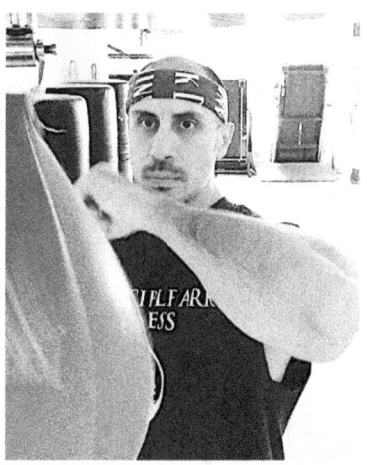

CROSS-TRAINING

It's essential not to get caught up in just one phase of training, for example, performing the same form (kata) every day or a monotonous weightlifting routine. Most strength and conditioning coaches recognize that it's beneficial to incorporate cross-training methods such as playing different sports, strength training, speed exercises, aerobics, calisthenics, plyometrics, isometric exercises, or other martial arts.

Learning a weapon can enhance body connection and footwork to execute your techniques more proficiently. Also, training weapons are great for improving your grip, which is beneficial for styles that use a gi or kimono, like judo and jiu-jitsu.

Cross-training is vital because life is unpredictable and at any moment you may need to run, jump, squat, lift, or fight, and the body must always be at its peak and ready for action no matter what. If you are not well-rounded in different areas of cross-training, you may have miscues in timing and performance that may deter you from successful outcomes in certain functions with which your body is not familiar.

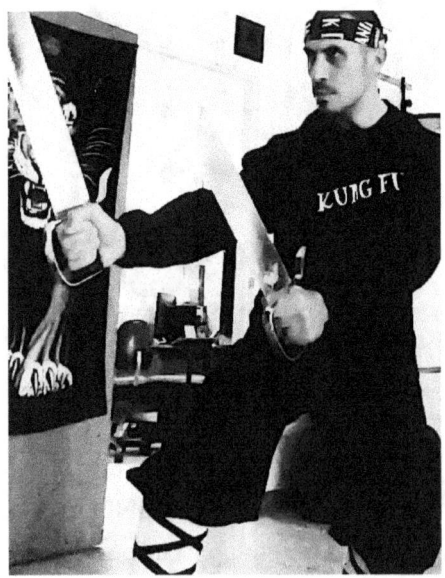

It's critical to maintain our overall physical conditioning because the world and people are unpredictable, and a confrontation could be around the corner later today, or even when you sleep. One of the warrior codes is "expect the unexpected," which takes self-discipline and plenty of self-sacrifice.

Struggle is nature's way of strengthening a living thing; therefore, the harder an individual trains, the better the results. Still, there must be boundaries because overtraining can damage your results. For this reason, please understand the cause, which is to know yourself and your limitations.

Elite warriors produce tremendous power and move quickly and effortlessly with fluidity. Consider the revered power-generating fighters of this generation and those prior—the most common characteristic they share is <u>consistently practicing the basics and fundamentals</u>. Furthermore, each practitioner is or was well-rounded, with the specific attributes and skills required for their craft.

Every martial art has distinctive movements that require specific routines to achieve proficiency. Also, there are strength and conditioning exercises specific to each martial art that enhance performance. All of these require motor learning for that particular style, technique, or activity, which takes time and persistent effort to convert to skilled performance.

Just because you are proficient in one style does not mean that your proficiency will automatically transfer to another training method. For example, you may have an excellent ground game but lack the agility for striking (or vice versa), or you may have spent years practicing Karate but struggle with the non-traditional footwork that Filipino martial arts use for speed and angled attacks.

Every single movement, technique, or exercise administers correctly through awareness of detail. You can deliver a precise performance if you practice your skills successfully and exhibit the factors of power, speed, endurance, and agility when executing them.

THE MIND-BODY CONNECTION

The brain and body are connected through the cerebrospinal system of nerves. The actions of thinking, processing, acting and reacting are all parts of a neuromuscular procedure we call the **mind-body connection**.

In combat, a warrior calls on muscle memory to execute the desired action through two avenues:

1. **The cerebrospinal system**, which is the avenue of the conscious "awakened" mind that receives perceptions and utilizes control over the movements of the body.
2. **The sympathetic nervous system** (different from the cerebrospinal system) is the avenue of the subconscious "habit" mind. This means the mental action we gain through our habits unconsciously supports the required functionality of the body.

Regardless of the technical process, the preparation of motor skills required for particular bodily movements or actions begins and ends with the work and habits we attain from constant physical practice.

The best way to prepare for unpredictable situations is to not overwhelm yourself with too much information. Instead, consistently focus on one set of moves that are second nature. Sometimes, when you "know too much," this can backfire when you try to transfer the knowledge into action.

Our opponent could overwhelm us, or smash us, and this can create negative or destructive thoughts due to our emotions. If we panic or get too sensitive to this kind of stress, it can hurt our agility and ability to react, causing us to make stupid mistakes in the moment. To avoid this happening, sparring is a significant factor in conditioning both our mind and body. The more a practitioner persists under stressful situations, the more agile and reactive they will become under duress.

According to Dan Inosanto, Bruce Lee was renowned amongst his peers as being excellent at sparring due to his ability to remain calm and collected, which he gained from the experience of sparring often. This poise enabled him to read his opponents' bodily movements to help him anticipate their next move.

WE ALL NEED A GOOD COACH

It's important to note that practice does not necessarily make perfect, because if you're practicing incorrectly, the technique loses its effectiveness. To avoid this, condition your subconscious mind with the proper technique, which is ensured by **the reasoning will**‡‡ of the conscious mind.

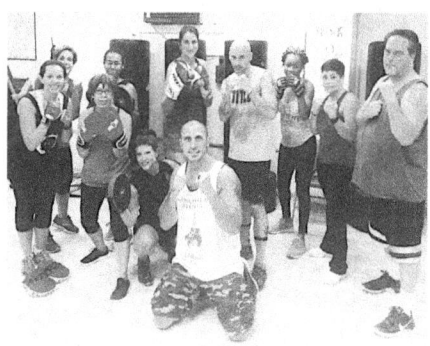

Change is inevitable, so resist rigidity and be willing to adapt to change. We are all constantly evolving. Even when you learn something new, you are replacing old information. When you age, gain or lose weight, grow taller, or get stronger, it's difficult to establish the precise motor skills needed, so your

---

‡‡ The ability to understand something and choose between whether it's correct or wrong, and whether it can be improved upon; yet having the determination to act upon that choice.

neuromuscular system can interfere with your performance. This constant change is why you need a good coach. Remember I asked you in the third chapter: *who is your master?*

Presently, most people want to teach what "they know," and in this information age, they tend to act like they know everything. Although most coaches relay what they have learned through their lineage or family tree, this doesn't necessarily mean they know how to train others.

A quality instructor knows how to develop new skills and abilities during these changing periods. If the coach fails to be creative or adapt to change, it forces a lot of martial artists to leave the system and move on.

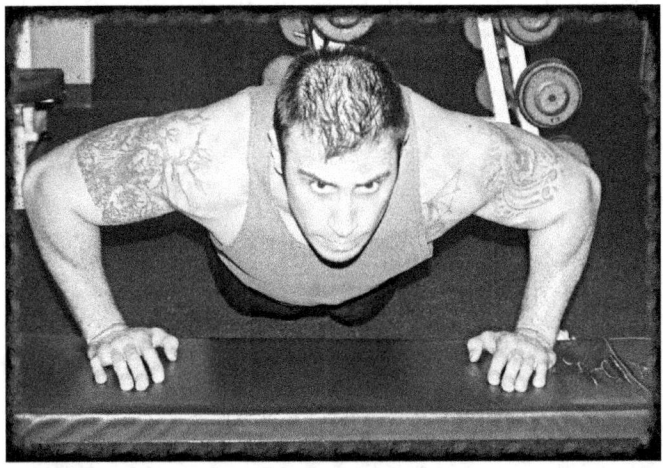

It's challenging to train everyone in the same way. Some may have reached their ceiling, which their coach must help them break through otherwise they may regress or lose interest. The opposite may be true as well, and a practitioner may be too slow to progress or have many limiting factors. The coach has to see and feel the energy of each student and be aware of everyone's skill level to provide the proper stimulation during training.

If you ever become a coach, never stop learning, training, and evolving—otherwise, everyone will drain your energy and you will have none left for yourself.

It takes years to integrate changes in motor skills into execution, especially since the central nervous system is continuously adapting to the changes of the muscular system and the **metabolism**, which is the core component in overall body performance.[44]

Those who wish to master the body must understand the importance of metabolism and that without energy from it, there would be no such thing as a movement. Still, regular and vigorous exercise combined with the proper diet creates the best opportunities to develop metabolic health to maintain and procure optimal energy. *So, how do we get to that level?*

As you progress, you start to change, your energy production increases, and your **internal electricity**[§§] grows stronger. A good coach identifies all of the elements that can make you better, link them together, and design them in a motor program specifically for you. This way, all of your moves may coordinate smoothly, and you may progress towards betterment as you grow.

Coaching takes skill. Most coaches use a combination of partial and whole methods to teach martial arts. Instruction in small parts allows the student to identify the components that make up the entire technique, whereas the whole method approach is best for simple skills like a punch or a kick. All of the problematic abilities are learned and become beneficial when taught alternatively by way of both methods.

The motor skills needed for martial art techniques are highly specific, and working on parts of any motion or action is only a fraction of the whole move or the "big picture." For this reason, it's important that a coach helps you integrate each movement into full fluidity, as this enables you to progress faster. Practicing

---

§§   Internal electricity: Qi force

the components of any action is *never* the same as performing the entire motion at full capacity. This is why sparring is vital.

ATHLETIC AGILITY

In martial arts, every style has particular exercises passed down through its lineage that produce a specific agility for that style. The x-factor is that we each have distinct builds and different athleticism. Each applied drill requires persistence from the practitioner to absorb them, especially when most exercises are either awkward or painful in the beginning.

It's beneficial to choose drills that will enhance your coordination and agility skills. Agility is the ability to move or change directions rapidly, which requires coordination. When your conscious mind practices them, your subconscious mind retains them and they become a fixed habit. All skills require the practitioner to be agile, which comes with time, patience, and hard work.

Some styles such as boxing, kung fu, and kali increase your coordination tremendously due to their awkward movements. They enable you to acquire agility and translate that agility into natural movements once learned. As most martial arts require directional change such as side-stepping or angulation, a practitioner needs to adjust their movements progressively so the body position can change rapidly and accelerate when necessary. Agility plays a significant role in this transition.

A good coach consistently emphasizes the correct movements, helping to eliminate bad habits and incorrect methods, especially when practicing at full speed. When the technique is right, then agility improves. To have coordination during execution, you need to prepare in basic fundamental techniques such as footwork and stance training. It's the transition from being rooted in your stance to becoming light on your feet that makes the difference. Practicing basic footwork will produce rapid and agile movements in combat. Footwork helps you win fights, so please understand that **athleticism** plays a significant role in helping a martial artist generate power.

If you don't know how to condition the body, then connect with a strength and conditioning coach who does. A skilled coach understands how to minimize injury by taking the proper precautions in activity, especially when a student is exhibiting poor execution. These preventative measures require adequate coaching and instruction. When a coach is genuinely knowledgeable and dedicated to their students, they'll instruct students in the proper strength and conditioning methods that enhance skill, prevent injury, and invigorate the spirit.

Unfortunately, the majority of martial arts have been watered down due to Western business standards, where kids get participation trophies and become conveyor black belts in two years. In addition, many classic styles focus on forms (katas) with barely any practical application, and the results are apparent when people use it in combat and fail miserably.

A good coach who has taken the time and earned their knowledge is in a great position to help others evoke their inner warrior. However, the problem we often face is finding an exceptional coach who did not themselves come from a conveyor belt and believes that money is secondary to honor, integrity, and mutual benefit. They are rare, but if you do your research, you can find them.

FIERCE TIGER PUSHING THE MOUNTAIN

Training for power is never easy, primarily because acquiring it depends on genetics, metabolic energy, muscular strength, skill level, and the central nervous system's capacity for reaction.

A warrior interested in developing dynamic power for martial arts must find a **balance** between lifting weights, building core strength, and applying all of the specific strength and conditioning training methods in their daily routine.

Repetition is key, especially when practiced at maximum intensity. When the muscles are overloaded with work, it helps boost your power. Without power, there is only mediocrity, and this will become apparent when there is a lack of conviction and limited success behind your actions. The conflict or struggle is necessary to reach a higher level.

Power is what separates excellence from mediocrity. Size has nothing to do with power. A warrior can be any size or shape (Bruce Lee was 5'8" and 128lbs) and still exhibit powerful blows. This powerful impact occurs when utilizing the full body connection, which is engaged by the legs and delivered by the core. This delivery of energy happens when the central nervous system is trained to react quickly, and the practitioner has the skillset to deliver the movements smoothly using their neuromuscular coordination of total body synergy.

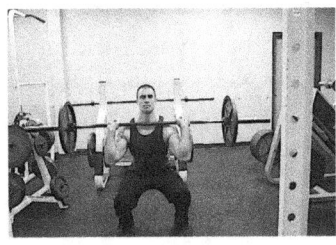 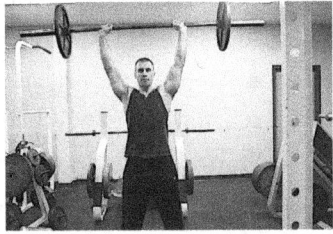

We measure power by the amount of work performed in a unit of time, which in essence is the energy that produces excessive force rapidly.[45] This process is why power and speed are synonymous with each other. Power is not based strictly on strength or speed; it is the combination of force from *both* attributes executed simultaneously. Developing speed and strength may increase your explosiveness, but it is the **synergistic movement** of the entire body that maximizes the delivery of a powerful technique.

Although it may take years to develop, learning how to execute a strike using the whole body synergistically with your legs, core, twisting of your hips, and upper body ensures the appropriate timing and connection to move fluidly.

Another aspect of conditioning needed to obtain power, especially for close-combat grappling, are the physical forces of **pushing** and **pulling**. The opposing forces of push and pull require excellent core strength using power driven by the legs. This is why kung fu stance training is vital, along with the majority of weight training exercises, including pulls, presses, deadlifts, squats, and core twists. These will benefit any practitioner greatly, so that the execution of each grab, lock, twist, trip, sweep, push, and throw is **dynamic**.

When we *combine* speed training with weightlifting, general conditioning, and skill development, a warrior is born—one sure to be quick in their delivery. Speed isn't just limited to offensive attacks, but also elusive footwork such as jumping, slipping, dodging, weaving, blocking, and other evasive measures to procure a great defense.

To develop speed, you need **repeated intensity** to enhance your capacity for acceleration. There are times when a martial artist needs to let go by removing all boundaries to improve the speed of a technique. If a practitioner has the mobility to move efficiently and follow through on all of the methods, then the skills will not only be **swift** and **explosive**, but **deadly**.

To improve mobility (which helps the body move more efficiently), aerobics and plyometrics[¶¶] are vital components that develop speed and explosiveness for performance, especially

---

[¶¶] Jumping exercises where muscles exert maximum force in short intervals of time.

during combat. Aerobics play an integral role in training because they increase your body's ability to transport oxygen. Aerobic capacity is a necessity, as it means more than just a healthy heart or fit body. **Aerobic exercise is what sets one martial artist apart from the rest.** It's beneficial to increase your stamina because fatigue turns a warrior into a coward. Strength, speed, and even power are ineffective without the **stamina** to fulfill them.

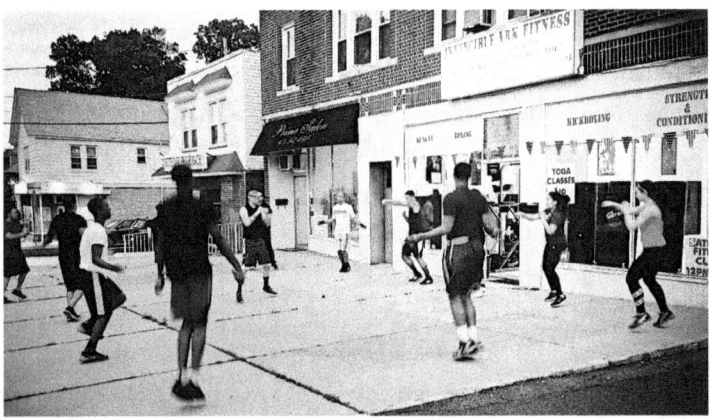

There is no quitting; continue to persist until the work or conflict is complete. **Endurance** is a necessary characteristic for all martial artists. If you don't have the staying power needed for combat, then you won't last very long in a fight. Warriors need to incorporate some form of cardiovascular exercise into their training. Basic aerobic exercises that are perfect for martial artists are jogging, running, climbing stairs, and jumping rope.

The best results come from training these exercises in intervals, such as **high-intensity interval training** (HIIT).[46] Use interval training to enhance the central nervous system's reaction time. This also helps the body's cells to endure rapid changes in metabolism and energy conduct.

STRONG AS AN OAK

When it comes to strengthening the body, focus on *all* of it, because there are many natural weapons you can use in combat to be effective (i.e. your head, shoulders, elbows, forearms, hands, knees, shins, and feet). All your limbs need strengthening to be useful. To condition these body parts correctly, you need to expose them to repeated strikes in sparring, partnered conditioning drills, iron palm bags, heavy bags, focus mitts, and a *mook jong* (a martial arts wooden dummy).

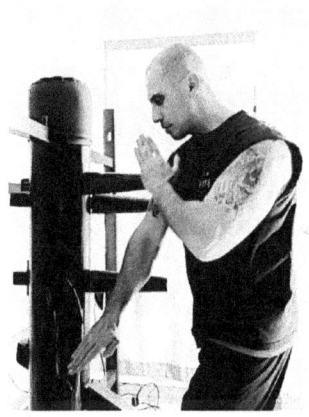

Having the ability to **endure punishment or take a hit** is vital. Whether you're training for sport or combat, your nerves and bones as well as your mind need conditioning. When we hit, we must not feel it or when we get hit, let it stun us so drastically that it makes us emotional, thereby losing our focus. When we are punched or kicked, we accept it as a natural part of combat. Also, while under duress or getting smashed, we must not lose our composure, stop breathing, or turtle up. We must keep moving forward.

Strengthening our muscles is incomplete without hardening our bones, which make up the primary structure of the body.

Conditioning our bones using the proper tools and partnered striking techniques will desensitize the nerve endings in the body and decrease the feeling of any impact.

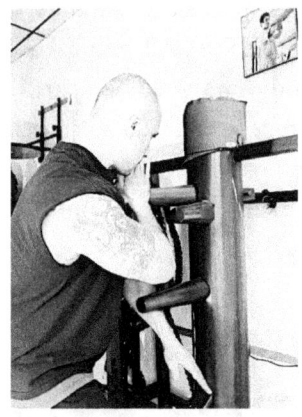

You may also need the medicine of **wine liniments**, known as *dit-da jow*. This natural healing method has been used by Chinese doctors and herbalists for centuries to help heal bruises, and is made of herbs and roots. You can order these online or find them at a pharmacy in your local Chinatown.

Conditioning begins with your forearms and shins, which are bridges to your opponent. Your forearms and legs must be as strong as an oak. Not only do you have to build the forearm and leg muscles until they are robust, but it's best if they continue to clash against other forearms, or the *mook jong*.

It's also beneficial to desensitize the nerve endings in your shins, which are very sensitive. Apply rolling and tapping methods with wooden dowel rods, and repeatedly kick heavy bags. You can work with a partner to lightly tap each other's shins (shin to shin) and kick each other's thighs to make them stronger, plus practicing the three-star blocking method*** (*da saam sing*) for the forearms and iron palm training for the hands.

***   Instructional videos for this drill can be found on YouTube.

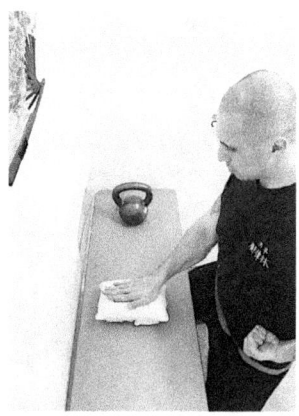

Hand to hand toss and catch with the iron palm bag is great for improving your tiger claw grip, which is beneficial for hand-locking styles like kung fu (chin na) and kali, and styles that use a gi or kimono, like judo and jiu-jitsu.

Although these conditioning methods are effective, <u>practice them with caution</u>. Experienced practitioners warn against overdoing this type of conditioning, due to consequences they faced later on in life. You will know you're overtraining if you experience constant pain.

In particular, condition your head with extreme caution due to the severity of concussion. Headgear is a useful tool here. However, please understand that on the streets or in a cage, there is no headgear. To adequately prepare, you must know what it feels like to get punched or kicked in the head; please use headgear regardless. Otherwise, the shock will either knock you out or diminish your confidence in the moment, making you want to quit. Once you tap out mentally, it's over for you physically.

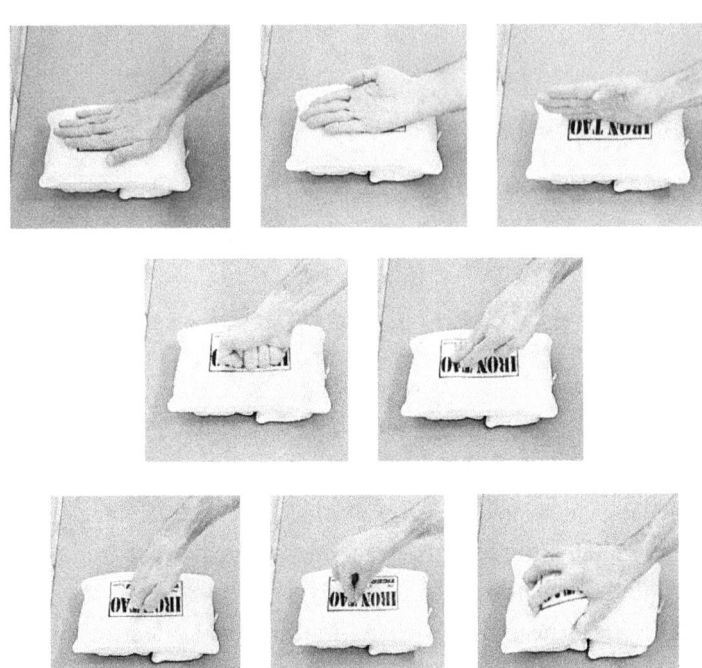

TWO TIGERS HIDE THEIR TRACKS

When we disobey nature's rules or try to force a particular outcome, her laws hold us back from growth, development, and success. This means that a warrior finds a balance between exercise and recovery. Activity is physical, and healing is mental. If the pain of training becomes intolerable, then why continue? Everything we do to become the best version of ourselves must make us stronger both physically and mentally—and in a positive manner, which means enjoying the process and severing the ties with negative emotions and destructive results.

Excessive training can cause injuries, anxiety, weight loss, insomnia, depression, chronic muscle soreness, and delayed recovery. All martial arts require an inherent love and passion for them, which means that any practitioner makes training fun and enjoyable. If you lose sight of the joy and pleasure that you gain from physical and mental stimulation during training—as well as your personal growth in the attainment of knowledge and wisdom—this will create negativity within you.

There are times in your training when you may push your body over the edge, and it might start reminding you of your limitations through pain, injury and sickness. At this point, resting your body becomes more important than working out.

Rest is always essential for warriors, especially since you won't make significant gains without adequate rest. Sometimes, rest is just as important as exercise, because it helps the body heal from hard work and improves overall fitness level.

A warrior remains headstrong and disciplined so the body may follow. No matter what happens, stay positive, stay strong, and stay focused on administering your training plan. The best method is to start slowly. I know that everyone wants to go quickly, but slow and steady wins the race.

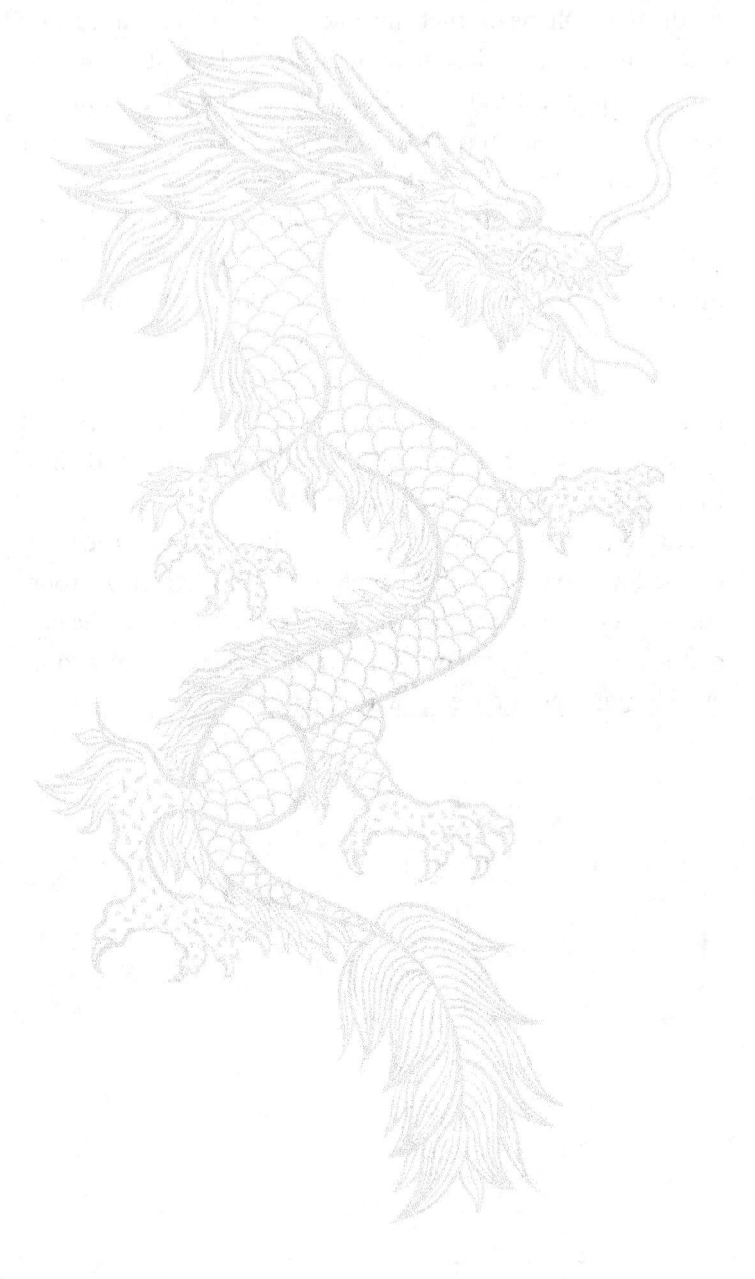

CHAPTER 9: NUTRITION

"The first wealth is good health."

— Ralph Waldo Emerson[47]

Good health contributes towards a **positive mental attitude**, meaning optimism, constructive behavior, precision in thoughts, decision making, and attributes such as agility and coordination.

The body is a sacred temple and an apparatus for power. I believe that it is one of the most miraculous instruments ever created and is a gift that our beloved Creator bestowed upon us. The human body is a remarkable illustration of **omnipotent architecture**, not just for the sole reason that it houses our consciousness, but because it is self-maintaining and a conductor of heat, electricity, frequency, and vibration.

The body requires **energy**, so what you put into it is what you will get out of it. If your ultimate purpose in life is obtaining power, then you need to feel your best in every moment. That's hard to do if you're always sick or nursing an injury. So, if you want to infuse yourself with positive energy, practice sound nutrition. If not, you will end up with pain, sickness, lack of focus, imbalances, weakness, sluggishness, and an inability to perform when needed.

Energy comes from the food we consume by way of vitamins, minerals, proteins, fats, carbohydrates, and water. These six nutrients are vital for the body to run efficiently, and they determine the functionality of our metabolism.

In life, most of our health issues reside through a lack of proper nutrition. Nutritional deficiency is a significant cause of physical sickness and mental anxiety. The key to nutrition is food, which in essence is fuel. It's crucial for our health and performance because it provides nutrients for our tissues and cells. Therefore, it's imperative to learn about and understand food to get the best results for your daily life.

When you know how to eat, what to eat, and when to eat, this provides a clear understanding of how much fuel you need to perform. This information is important for individuals who want to practice healthy, disciplined eating habits. The level of strictness depends on the individual, but sensible eating can help anyone achieve their goals.

Carbohydrates are the body's main fuel source for performance energy. Therefore, our capacity for any action and mental processing diminishes quickly when we're low on carbs. There are two forms of carbohydrates: simple and complex. Complex carbs are more important for an athlete or martial artist because they provide energy for high-performance training. The body usually converts these carbs into energy, but consuming more than you expend leads to excessive body fat.

Ideal complex carbs for athletes:[48]
- Oatmeal
- Fruits
- Sweet potatoes
- Whole wheat and ancient grain pasta
- Brown and wild rice

When your muscles break down or are atrophied (wasted), your body needs **protein** to repair and replenish them. Proteins are constructed of **amino acids**, and are necessary because they provide the structural material that composes all of our muscle tissue, bones, enzymes, hormones, and cell membranes. We need adequate protein because it contributes to the physical requirements necessary for training and combat, but also because it helps to replenish muscle tissue afterward. As such, it plays a critical role in muscle recovery.

Fats are the most energy-rich food source for the body. Fat is necessary for the body because it's a storage depot for energy. Fats insulate and protect the internal organs. However, too much fat is unhealthy and negates speed, endurance, and power.

As you can see, good nutrition is essential for health and performance, and is one of the primary methods to obtain physical strength. It's significant in providing you with the energy needed to perform at a higher level. Furthermore, the conversion of food to fuel for muscular endurance determines our levels of performance. For example, poor nutrition may enable an unhealthy or obese person to be explosive for an action or two (although it may be slow and predictable), but after that, they may fall apart quickly.

MONKEY STEALS A PEACH

Humans obtain energy through foods, liquids, or supplements. However, just because you ingest certain foods and liquids, this doesn't automatically transform them into useful energy. It's helpful to understand that high-energy foods will lead to vitality and a longer, healthier life.

For example, we can fight fatigue and oxidative stress[†††] by consuming high-quality calories, especially from fruits and vegetables, to restore the energy levels in our muscles and liver.

---

††† Oxidative stress is an imbalance between free radicals and antioxidants in the body, which can lead to cell and tissue damage.

Eating a well-balanced ratio of food that mostly consists of fruits and vegetables will provide the sixteen essential vitamins and minerals that your body needs to keep up with daily physical maintenance.

Unfortunately, no single fruit or vegetable contains all of these vitamins and minerals, so it's vital to eat a variety of fruits and vegetables. If you lack the required nutrients, you can buy a raw whole-food supplement derived from natural food sources. These give you the health-building factors essential for wellbeing. When you metabolically convert an array of fruits and vegetables into energy, you gain the power of nature.

ALKALINIZATION

"No disease, including cancer, can exist in an alkaline environment."

— Dr. Otto Warburg[49]

Otto Heinrich Warburg was born in Germany, 1883. He was a physiologist and medical doctor, receiving his doctorate in chemistry in 1906 and medicine in 1911. He became well-known for his research called "The Chemical Constitution for Respiration Ferment" in 1928. In this research, he differentiated between the energy consumption of regular cells versus cancer cells in the body.[50]

In 1931, Warburg received the Nobel Prize in Physiology or Medicine for his work in discovering the nature and mode of action of the respiratory enzyme. His scientific research on the aerobic and anaerobic metabolic processes in cells, and the metabolism of tumors and respiration of cells (particularly cancer cells) was revolutionary. It still holds true today, especially in what we know about cancer.

Based on his findings, I believe that it's beneficial to nourish your body with alkaline foods. There is plenty of mixed information out there on this topic, but I have found that more doctors are starting to incorporate a holistic approach to health with alternative medicines and nutrition plans.

Of course, I urge everyone I coach to consult with their physician or a nutritionist. Please do some research and study the fruits and vegetables that are beneficial and restore the body's pH level. An alkaline state neutralizes the whole body, which helps to keep it balanced.

ALKALINE FOODS: Almonds, Amaranth, Apple Cider Vinegar (with the root known as "the mother"), Artichokes, Arugula, Asparagus, Avocado, Basil, Beetroot, Broccoli, Brussels Sprouts, Buckwheat, Cabbage, Carrots, Cauliflower, Celery, Chia Seeds, Chives, Cilantro, Coconut, Collard Greens, Cucumber, Cumin, Dandelion Greens, Eggplant, Endives, Garlic, Flax Seeds, Ginger, Grapefruit, Graviola, Green Beans, Green Tea, Kale, Kelp, Khorasan Wheat, Leek, Lemons, Lentils, Lettuce, Lima Beans, Lime, Mint, Mung Beans, Navy Beans, Okra, Olive Oil, Onions, Parsley, Peas, Peppers, Pomegranate, Pumpkin, Quinoa, Radishes, Red Beans, Rhubarb, Sesame Seeds, Spinach, Squash, Sunflower Seeds, Sweet Potato, Swiss Chards, Thyme, Watercress, Wheatgrass, White Tea, and Zucchini to name a few.

The earth provides nutritious fruits and vegetables, which hold most of the nutrition required by human beings in an easily digestible form. The ancient Chinese masters of Shaolin[51] believed that a vegetarian diet helped to generate the body's Qi energy and allowed the thermal force to move quickly throughout the body and its energy hubs known as **chakras**[52] (these stem from Hindi beliefs).

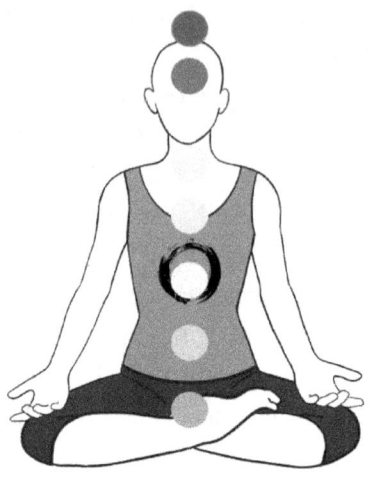

According to the ancient belief system of traditional Chinese medicine[53] practiced by acupuncturists[54] for over two thousand years, when this flow occurs, all of the body's meridians[‡‡‡] are open and there are no blockages to stop the flow of energy. This natural progression of blood and energy is essential to balance the mind-body connection.

However, not just the ancient masters promoted this diet. Even the American Academy of Nutrition and Dietetics[55] states that it's beneficial to follow vegetarian eating habits and reduce or eliminate the consumption of meat. According to the Harvard Medical School's special health report *Healthy Eating: A guide to the new nutrition*,[56] there are pros and cons to becoming a vegetarian, yet it provides many health benefits such as:

1. Reduced bad cholesterol
2. Reduced inflammation
3. Lower blood pressure
4. Lower body mass index (BMI)

[‡‡‡] Paths or channels in the body through which the life-energy known as "qi" flows.

5. Reduced risk of heart disease
6. Reduced risk of developing certain cancers
7. Reduced risk of acquiring Type-2 Diabetes

These resources and the International Sports Sciences Association advise that you can make your meals mostly vegetarian without going all the way.[57] For example, the Mediterranean diet consists of mostly plant-based foods with a moderate intake of lean meats such as fish and chicken, and healthy fats like olive oil.

The Mediterranean eating style is well-known throughout the fitness industry due to its association with reduced chronic illnesses and longer life spans. Regardless, the most important factor in nutrition is finding what works best for you by consulting a physician or nutritionist.

TRADITIONAL CHINESE MEDICINE DETOXIFICATION

When a human being is nutritionally out of balance, they may experience illness or injury, and decide to resort to narcotics and pharmaceutical drugs. However, all this does is negate their power even further, and makes everything worse for both the mind and body. I know this from my own personal experiences with alcohol and painkillers.

With that said, many circumstances affect the production of qi energy, especially with regard to brain functionality. Qi doesn't respond well to bad foods, alcohol, and drugs because these are unnatural substances that harm the body and disrupt the blood, heart, liver, kidneys, and brain.

There is a collective ignorance, especially in the Western world, around liver and kidney care. This neglect has led to various illnesses and dependencies on pharmaceutical medication for people to function daily.

According to Dr. Sandra Cabot,[58] excessive amounts of certain medicines (such as antihistamines, cimetidine, and antidepressants) tend to damage the liver and decrease its ability to extract nutrients from food, eliminate toxic poisons, as well as eliminating heavy metals from the bloodstream.

This is supported by WebMD,[59] and case studies from the National Center of Biotechnology Information (NCBI)[60] based on tests from the U.S. National Institute of Health's National Library of Medicine (NIH, NLM).[61] These studies showed that particular nonsteroidal anti-inflammatory drugs (NSAIDs) can increase disease and toxicity in the liver. Furthermore, a study from the University of South Alabama College of Medicine[62] along with the Food and Drug Administration[63] state that over the counter (Tylenol) and prescription painkillers (i.e. Percocet, Vicodin) all contain high doses of acetaminophen, which can increase the risk of liver damage.

All of the internal organs are directly connected to the brain. However, some traditional medicine doctors (such as Sandra Cabot),[64] traditional Chinese medicine practitioners, and homeopathic medicine theory (especially in the field of Anthroposophy), believe the liver is the second most vital organ next to the brain. The liver is a sponge that filters everything that passes through the body. Your liver is the body's front-line defense against harmful toxins. When you take care of your liver, your brain becomes sharper and helps to fight any harmful toxins that attack the body. Therefore, it's critical to keep the liver and intestines clean and orderly to increase mental clarity and feel good.

As the liver and brain are directly related, care for both to ensure they function properly. It's essential to provide the liver with supplementation to release toxins and antioxidants for detoxification, improving physical and mental health, and circulation. You can use special herbs, roots, seeds, and barks, such as milk thistle,[65] chicory seeds,[66] yarrow,[67] Arjuna bark,[68] tamarisk,[69] dandelion,[70] and graviola[71] to name a few.

When the body's systems are clogged and stagnant, the flow of elimination ceases and this subdues the body with low energy and physical and mental instability.

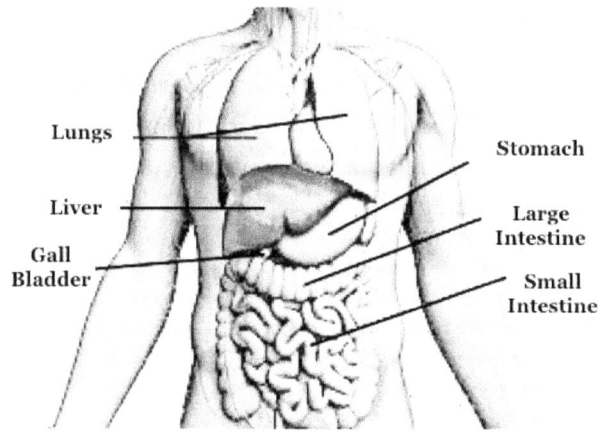

Bowel movements are crucial to the body's vitality. Anyone who eats wisely and keeps their elimination system clean may have a healthier flow in their digestive tract.[72] This ensures exceptional brain functionality and the healthy function of all the internal organs.

Maintaining the internal organs is necessary to keep the inner body healthy. Please take care of your liver, kidneys, and intestines and try to avoid narcotics and pharmaceutical drugs. This may not resonate with you now, but as you grow older, it will. You can maintain your vitality as you age, and this begins by not neglecting your wellbeing. Please understand that when your nutrition is correct, the need for medication may no longer exist.

THE POWER OF NATURE

"Let food be thy medicine, and medicine be thy food."

— Hippocrates[73]

According to Dr. Richard Schulze, one of the world's foremost authorities on natural healing and herbal medicine, **the entire human body rebuilds itself in less than two years.** In his clinical findings, he proclaims the following eight positions:[74]

1. The human body heals or regenerates itself by 98% in less than one year.[§§§]
2. The brain in one year.
3. The blood in four months.
4. The skeleton in three months.
5. The DNA in two months.
6. The liver in six weeks.
7. The skin in one month.
8. The stomach lining in five days.

In my personal experience, the body functions properly when you provide it with the ingredients to do so. Therefore, you must give your body proper nutrition and exercise. Nature provides all of the medicine you need for the maintenance of good health. She stores them in fruits, vegetables, whole grains, herbs, roots, and seeds.

There are some beliefs that different parts of the body regenerate in anywhere from a couple of days to seven years[75] according to carbon-14 dating generated by nuclear bomb tests during the

---

§§§ In a study published in the Annual Report for Smithsonian Institution in 1953, scientists found that 98% of our atoms are replaced each year.

Cold War (Dr. Jonas Frisen).[76] Various beliefs circulate on the internet, but if this is true, then it is our fault if we are subject to poor physical conditions year after year and continue to maintain the same body because of our bad habits.

It's my belief that the idea of overcoming our unfavorable conditions begins with resolutions. It's common knowledge that throughout the fitness industry, there is a spike in sales after the New Year, but within two to three months into the year, sales dip drastically. With the knowledge of our body's ability to heal itself, if you resolve to truly change at the beginning of the year, then by the end of that year, your conditions and results will more than likely change for the better.

Of course, everyone is built differently and there may be limiting factors in injury and illness prevention or recovery. For example, there are people who smoke cigarettes, drink alcohol, use narcotics, and eat all of the rich desserts they like, yet live long lives. Then there are people like Bruce Lee who never drank alcohol, exercised daily, ate a healthy diet, and died from a cerebral edema at thirty-two-years old. Regardless of our individual differences, I strongly believe that it's still important to practice healthy eating, because life is not about the way you die—it's about the way you live.

In the past, most of our ancestors ate to survive. In the present, many people eat for pleasure, stuffing different combinations of fatty foods, rich desserts, meats, dairy products, and excessive alcohol into their bodies, and these overwork the organs and complicate digestion.

When people ingest food in mass quantities, it overworks their heart, liver, kidneys, and intestinal tract. This can lead to elimination problems and other illnesses such as abdominal pain, blood in the stool, bloating, inflammation, constipation, diarrhea, nausea, vomiting, heartburn, and acid reflux. This is according to medical institutions such as the National Institute of Diabetes and Digestive and Kidney Diseases,[77] University of Texas MD Anderson Cancer Center,[78] and gastrointestinal studies from PubMed.[79]

It's ideal to control your thoughts and actions, so unless you're a wild animal or unsure where your next meal will come from, allow your body to digest food in smaller increments. It's destructive to overeat. Due to the overabundance of supply, and poor, undisciplined eating habits, it has become common for most people to overindulge with food and reap the side effects of weak body composition and excess belly fat.

Excess body fat relates to poor health and increases the risk of ongoing health problems. Although maintaining self-control and reducing body fat seem to remain a difficult task for most people, a disciplined warrior creates healthy eating habits no matter what.

To combat poor health and obesity, start with a healthy diet consisting of fruits, vegetables, whole grains, nuts, and olive oil. If you are a carnivore, stick to lean white meats or preferably fish (the Mediterranean diet). According to the National Institute of Health (NIH), eating red meat[80] and pork[81] has adverse effects on the body, can complicate your digestion, and may cause illness.

If you have to eat red meat, please limit it based on guidance from the United States Department of Agriculture (USDA).[82] It may be beneficial to eliminate pork entirely, because the Centers of Disease Control and Prevention (CDC),[83] National Institute of Health (NIH),[84] and a 2013 Consumers Report analysis state that the harmful parasites in pork (trichinella, tapeworm, and yersinia enterocolitica) stick to your intestines.[85]

Vegetarian animals are edible for human beings and may provide long-lasting energy, but that doesn't mean they are beneficial for your sustenance. The unfavorable treatment of such animals negates their real purpose and eventually catches up with us.

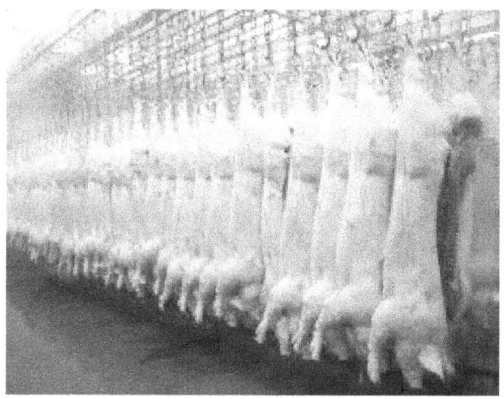

In today's society, most animals bred for food are ill-fed, mistreated, and abused. They are also injected with a variety of vaccines, drugs, antibiotics, and bovine steroids.[86] Their experience while living or dying is either fear or rage. As a consequence, they are filled with negative energy and develop cancer, which becomes harmful to the human body.[87]

The Shaolin belief is that the carnivorous diet negates the spiritual connection to all living things. The Shaolin monks believed that eating meat would give you the power and strength of that animal, so whatever it was, felt, and ate was the energy you would take upon yourself. But if the animal was sick, you could suffer too. If the animal felt fear, then you would feel anxiety as well.[88] These Buddhist beliefs stem from the Hindu belief system and are very similar to esoteric teachings and homeopathic/alternative medicine practices.

When you eat fruits and vegetables from the land, these foods will give you the power of nature. Nature's power is unlimited, and by eating the right foods, you can feel her immense power and energy. The choice is yours.

The following is a simple guide to help you on your quest to harness the power of nature through nutrition:
- **Raw organic fruits and vegetables** = the power of nature
- **Herbal supplementation** = the power of nature
- **Whole grains** = high fiber, digestion, lower cholesterol, and maintain low blood pressure
- **Olive oil** = healthy fats
- **Water** = the power of nature
- **Tea** = the power of nature
- **100% fruit and vegetable juice** = the power of nature
- **Meat** = the strength or weakness of the animal
- **Processed foods** = weak quality energy; empty calories
- **Soda** = poor quality energy; empty calories
- **Alcohol** = intoxication negates all power

Tea is beneficial for the body, especially after eating meals. Tea leaves are a gift from nature, and many different types offer a variety of benefits to help the human body digest and combat ailments. Seek them, understand them, and use them.

HUNGRY TIGER CATCHES THE LAMB

The rise of processed meat, fast food, French fries, processed sweets, and soft drinks has induced poor and imbalanced eating habits among the wider population.

According to Harvard Health, these fast foods have lead people to develop deadly toxic poisoning from food additives and chemicals, and develop various health risks (obesity, asthma, eczema, and more).[89] According to the World Cancer Research Fund (WCRF)[90] and the American Institute for Cancer (AIC),[91] these foods possibly even cause cancer. In 2018, an eight-year study showed that the people who followed their nutritional advice had a reasonably lower cancer risk, which was:[92]

- **Maintain a healthy weight:** Keep your weight within a healthy range and avoid weight gain in adult life.
- **Be physically active:** Be physically active as part of everyday life—walk and exercise more, sit less.
- **Eat wholegrains, vegetables, fruits, and beans:** Make them a major part of your usual diet.
- **Limit fast-foods:** Limit consumption of "fast-foods" and other processed foods high in fat, starches, and sugars.
- **Limit red and processed meats:** Eat no more than moderate amounts of red meat, such as beef, pork, and lamb. Eat little, if any, processed meats (avoid nitrates).
- **Limit sugar sweetened drinks:** Drink mostly water and unsweetened drinks.
- **Limit alcohol consumption:** For cancer prevention, it's best not to drink alcohol.
- **Don't rely on supplements:** Aim to meet nutritional needs through diet alone.

Most poor eating habits stem from ignorance and lack of self-control. The bulk of your diet must consist of fruits and vegetables. You should eat when you're hungry and eat healthy foods in between major meals instead of fast foods. The International Sports Sciences Association (ISSA) recommends minimizing your consumption of meats, butter, and grains such as bread, rice, pasta, potatoes, and sugar.[93]

In my opinion, sugar might be the devil of all foods. The following are just some of the negative effects of too much sugar in your diet according to PubMed:[94]

1. Obesity.
2. Type 2 diabetes.
3. Increased risk of heart disease.

4. Increased risk of various skin conditions (androgen secretion, oil production, inflammation, aging).
5. May increase your risk of cancer.
6. May increase your risk of declined dental health.
7. May increase your risk of kidney disease.
8. May increase your risk of depression.
9. Fatty liver.
10. Lower energy levels (sugar crash).

In life, you will benefit from understanding the principles and fundamentals of nutrition, being disciplined in your eating habits, and having total control of your food intake. This form of control empowers a warrior to sustain vitality, and a better quality of life.

GATE 2—KEY POINTS

1. Stay open-minded and receptive before reaching conclusions.
2. Learn about your body and master it before you try to help others.
3. Keep positive habits and carry them out persistently.
4. Strength is needed both internally and externally. Exercise the mind, body, and spirit vigorously.
5. Stretching is an integral part of circulation and feeling good.
6. Conditioning the body persistently helps to increase cell strength.
7. Nutrition is the key factor in overall health and wellness.
8. Detoxification is important to cleanse the body.
9. Sometimes, the rest is more important than the workout.
10. Find your weaknesses and strengthen them through persistence.

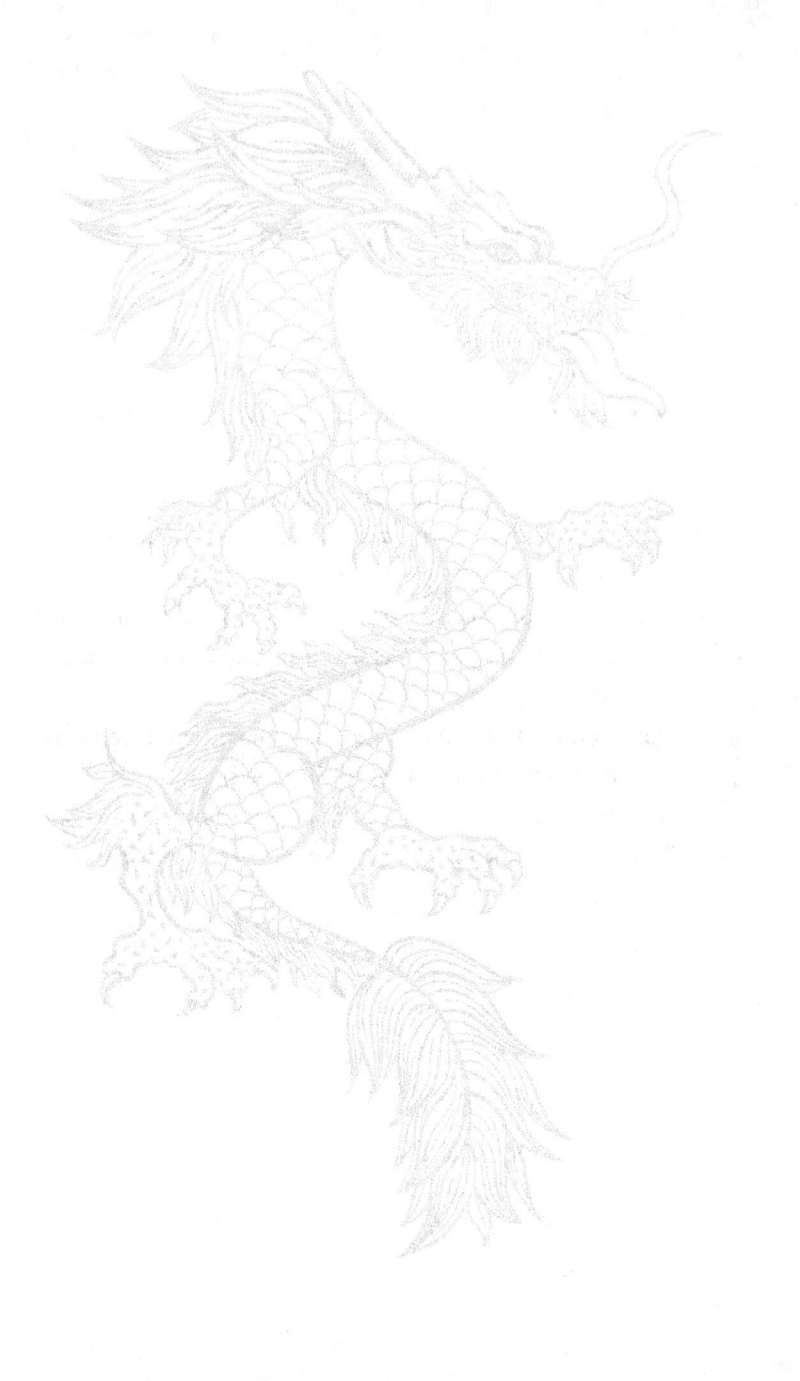

THE DRAGON

Everywhere in nature, there are circles of energy. The atmosphere, the earth, and the body all contain multiple rings of energy in different sizes. From the *enso* to the *ouroboros*, from people to circumstances, everything comes full circle.

The dragon is a treasure, not only because it is associated with wealth, good fortune, and rainfall for crops, but because once you face one, tame it, and harness its powers, the potential for its purpose is **infinite**. It's no wonder that most martial arts display the symbol of the dragon and use circles as a sigil. These disciplines embody the exploration of the true self who develops wisdom, creative imagination, and freedom to cultivate and deliver power.

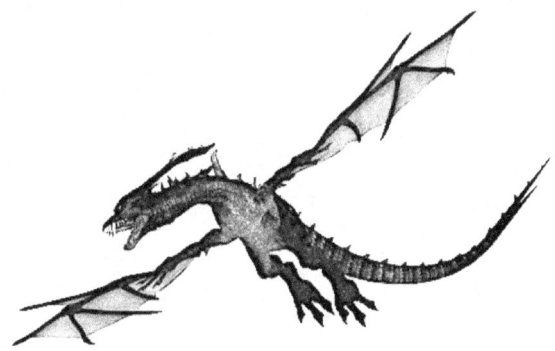

The dragon is alive in the heart of a warrior and inhabits the cave within the mountain. Only those who possess valor attempt to travel towards the interior to catch a glimpse of this magnificent beast. This enormous creature resides within the inner circle of the solar plexus and represents the unlimited potential that a human being possesses within.

Of all the animals in martial arts, the dragon reigns supreme because of its powerful ecliptic movements, coiling tendencies, and force of breath. Although the dragon delivers its potential in many ways, it harnesses and cultivates energy in a circular or spiraling fashion, similar to a double helix or the rolling waves of the ocean, which twist and turn into oblivion.

According to traditional Chinese medicine, our bodies are made up of internal **meridians**, just like the earth.[95] Our breathing cultivates energy and harnesses its power from our inner core. This cultivation of electricity, vibration, and heat all harmonize and balance the body perfectly. By using these special breathing skills, we can move heat into different parts of the body. This thermal transfer allows the practitioner to maintain stable health.

Finally, the dragon is strong and decisive. It knows its direction and purpose at all times. By thinking, breathing, and acting like a dragon, we obtain wisdom, confidence, and power in our delivery. The dragon is a circle and can break through all rings of power at any time. It is immovable and unbeatable. **The dragon is invincible,** and now, the third gate. . . .

GATE 3—INTERNAL ENERGY

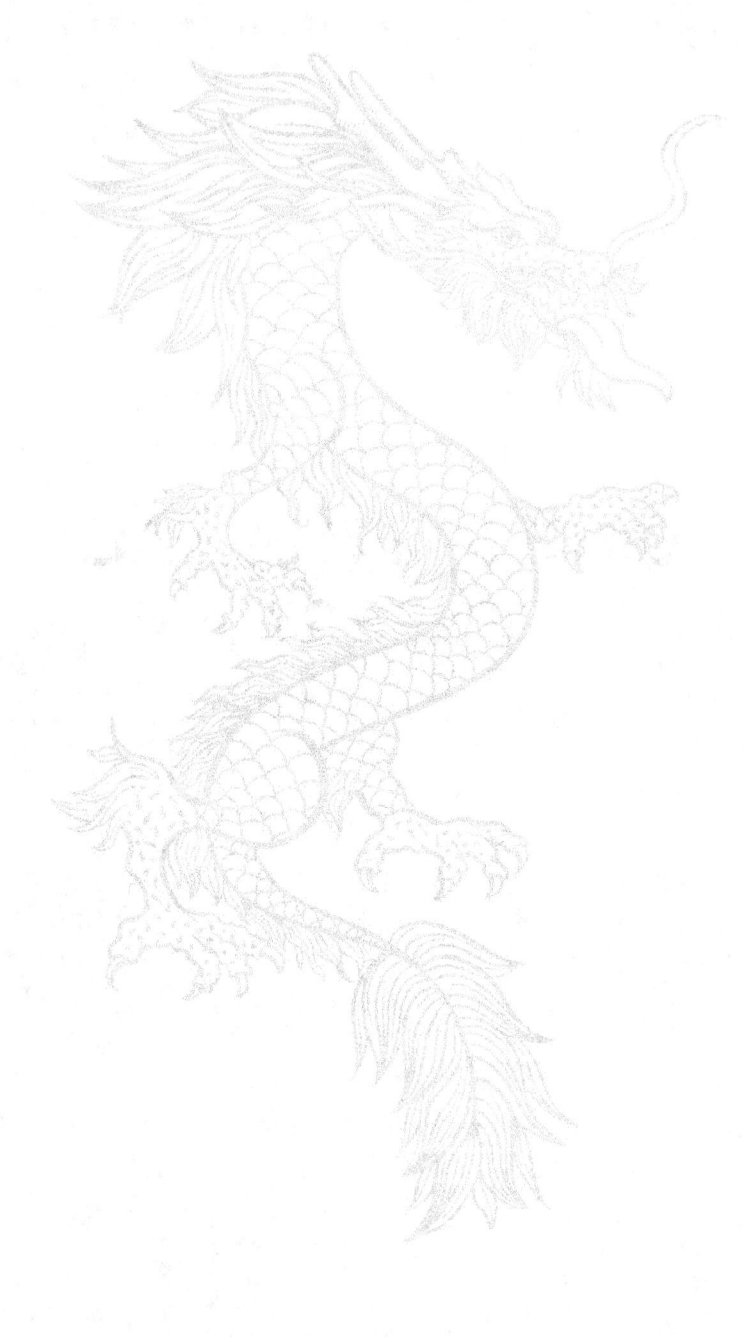

GATEWAY TO THE TEMPLE OF POWER

Welcome to the third gate towards invincibility. This gate will help you develop your body further and bring forth power-consciousness to connect both your mind and body in harmony to project energy and power.

Power is essential for success in any endeavor, especially in martial arts, and in the following chapters I will detail how the force of our internal energy plays a crucial role in our production, circulation, and expression of power. Please understand that all of the philosophies and techniques in martial arts are useless without sufficient power to transform them into action; therefore, power is a virtue that comes from within you. Most people look outwards for power, but the secret among masters is that you have to first look inside yourself, discover it, then develop it, and finally project it.

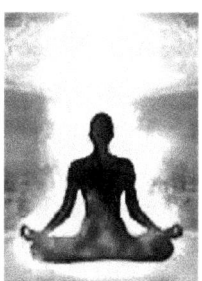

The warrior resides in two worlds. The first is **metaphysical**: the internal world; the inner realm of light; and the storehouse of power, home of the soul, and the subconscious mind. The second is the **physical**: the outside world; the outer realm of action and reaction; and the field of darkness or home of the body and the conscious reasoning mind.

The external world is a reflection of the internal world. What we find on the outside comes from the expressions we release from within. All power originates from the interior, the source of all energy, all wisdom, and all power. We are unable to express this power if we don't possess the mentality to discover and develop it. Also, we can't deliver any power if we don't obtain it first.

Internal power is an increase in the strength and energy within you. To generate it, always look within first, then go outwards. This relates to anything in life that you have to deal with, whether it's conflicts, work, relationships, or training. Most of the time, if a negative situation arises in life, it stems from your **thoughts, choices, actions,** or **reactions**. The way you think and act towards the situation depends on the internal power you have cultivated so far.

THE THREE POSITIONS OF POWER

What is the practicality of power? It is <u>the ability to elicit the favorable outcome you desire</u>. It requires both physical and metaphysical force, which is produced by the mind-body connection.

In our realm of existence, you will learn that we cultivate power from three different positions:

1. <u>SUPREME INTELLIGENCE</u>: Whether you call it Nature, Ether, God, Creator, or Source Energy, this is the ultimate authority of power that we interface with through our spiritual link found in the world within ourselves. The mental plane of consciousness in the world within is the storehouse of enormous energy. Energy is power, and Supreme Intelligence provides all of the energy and strength we need to attain power.

2. MINDS OF MAN: The accumulated experiences of other men and women, past and present, is organized and recorded in books and now on the internet. Although knowledge is forever evolving, any individual can easily attain information and expertise from masters and scholars online or in books to cultivate power. Under Supreme Intelligence, using men and women to relay messages of enlightenment, the world has obtained wisdom. You need this wisdom to grow and acquire power. When you become aware of this wisdom, you can use it to cultivate your abilities, and when you take possession of it, you can deliver it to the world around you.
3. PRACTICE: Our power ultimately comes from within. However, we must be aware of it before we can attain it. We crystallize our awareness and possession through research and experimentation, otherwise known as practice or action. When the experience matures, it becomes the **effect**. This raises our awareness to attain more power. Often, this occurs through the creative imagination. But to properly gain power, one must practice. No amount of accumulated hypothetical knowledge can ever substitute practice. Any plan is useless unless transformed into action and expressed with force. Regular practice creates a habit, inducing a response from the creative imagination, and so on. In other words, if you don't use it, you lose it. If you're not constructive, then you will never evolve, and plateaus are inevitable, which are the enemy of the martial artist.

These three methods are ways to attain power. In the following chapters, we will examine these three positions.

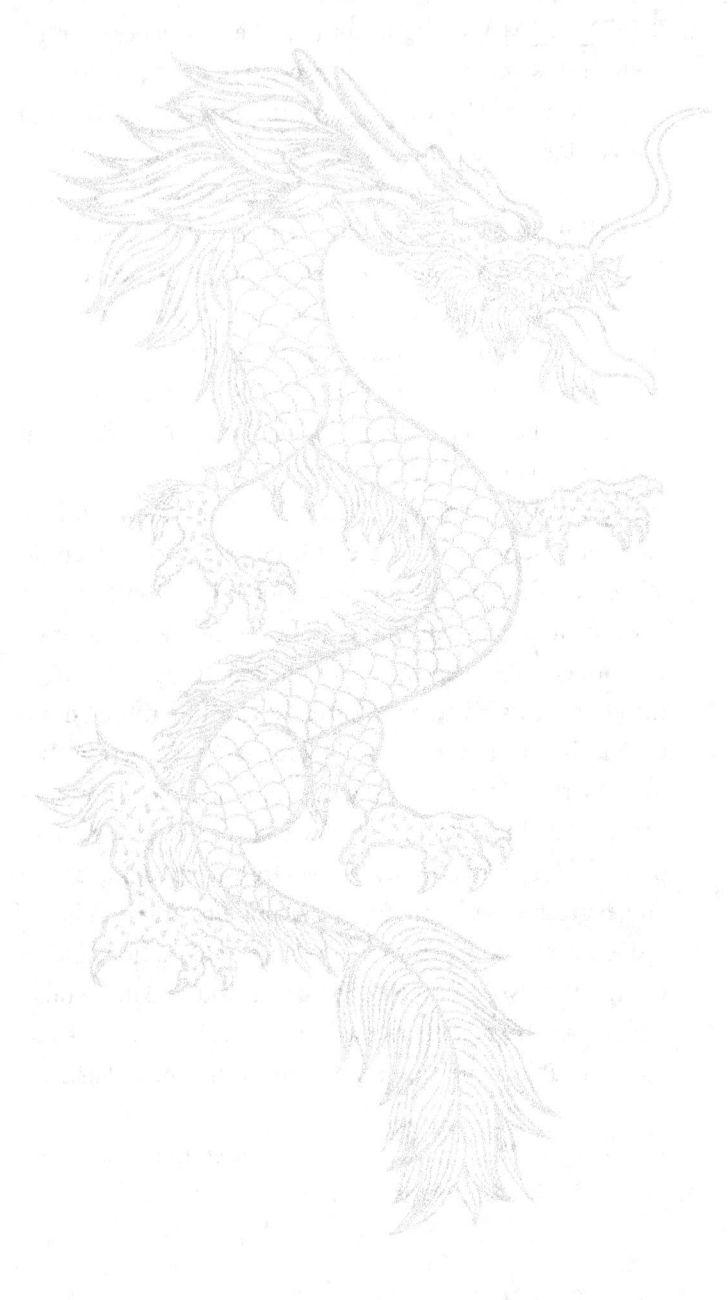

CHAPTER 10: POWER IN PROVIDENCE

I believe a monistic theory, the view that reality is one organic whole and there is only one ultimate substance. This theory that **all is one and one is all**, was passed down through the ages from great minds (Hermes, Pythagoras, Ralph Waldo Emerson, Wallace Wattles, Charles F. Haanel, and Manly P. Hall, among others), and is believed to stem from Hindu origins. The one life manifests itself as *everything*, every element, and every life in the physical world. This belief is the foundation for most Oriental philosophies.

Studying this philosophy in conjunction with training martial arts, I discovered the true power of the mind-body-spirit connection.

The **self** is part of this one life and is one with all life: the earth, the universe, the source of all energy and all power. This collective is part of a supreme intelligence, a universal mind, and this consciousness is believed by monists to be the creative force of the entire universe, which is a single living conscious organism with complete awareness of itself.

- **Ralph Waldo Emerson** said: "*Of the Universal Mind, each individual man is one more incarnation.*"[96]
- **Charles F. Haanel** stated: "*There is one principle or consciousness pervading the entire universe and all thoughts and things are within itself. It is all in all.*"[97]

- **Manly P. Hall** said: *"There is only one immutable divine force in the universe that gives life, vitality, energy, and opportunity to all living things. This one life is the only reason we are alive, without it, we could not even exist."*[98]

In *The Master Key System* (Charles F. Haanel, 1912), the conclusion is that the **one life** occupies all space and is essentially the same at every point of its existence.[99] From this, we can understand that this source is all-powerful, all-knowing, and always present. Therefore, the source of our internal power is the universal mind, otherwise known as this one life, the "all" in all.

We may get inspiration from this supreme intelligence that relays messages to us through the minds of other people, whether it's learning martial arts, practicing meditation, or gaining wisdom from books, but our power always comes from within the depths of our inner core. This is why it helps if you believe in yourself and your abilities, as this brings you clarity and depth of vision to attain the power you seek.

ONE LIFE

The first place that power comes to us from is **supreme intelligence**. Many masters, philosophers, and scholars agree that all is one and one is all. The one life in all is the first cause known as "**Providence**." Providence is, in other words, supreme intelligence.

According to monistic philosophy, this force is omnipotent (all-powerful), omniscient (all-knowing), and omnipresent (eternal).[100] This creative force is an energy that permeates **all matter, all space, and all time**. Many great thinkers and authors believe that this intelligence gives us the authority to think. Therefore, all thought is energy and an expression of the one life.

Our minds connect to this omnipotent force, which gives us the ability to think, and it is this comprehension that allows us to express ourselves as individuals, to crystallize the abstract energy from the spiritual realm into our physical plane of existence.

Energy is an expression of power, and Providence is the origin of the power that comes from within. Energy is the power to think, feel, create, and express specific actions, or in other words, have ideas, speech, actions, reactions, and sex.

In nature, the flow of energy is like a river, broken down into waves and currents that permeate every atom of matter. Providence uses this energy to construct everything in existence, including man, animal, vegetable, and mineral. The earth is our being and is made up of the hearts and minds of humanity. It is a reflection of our thoughts, providing all the power we need to harness and utilize more energy.

LIFT UP THE SKY AND COVER THE EARTH

Matter makes up everything in existence, and the energy that permeates every atom of matter is omnipotent, omniscient, and omnipresent. **We are all made of the same substance as the earth.** As a result, we are all one with the earth if we choose to be. When you can silence your mind and tap into the energy that flows within, you can feel and be one with the earth.

Infinite energy is all around us and sits deep within our bodies. Nature governs and balances all transactions and every force within us and around us to correspond with its origin: the one life, Providence.

The bond between the finite and the infinite is glued together by the atmosphere, which saturates the inner essence of our spirit. This power of nature is called the **ether**, and this fluid energy connects everything from people (their thoughts and actions) to everything else in existence.

The ether is a conduit for infinite power and allows an individual to experience life. The ether mirrors *now*, not the past, nor the future. The etheric reflection is the limitless power that we hold within us. The ether enables us to achieve the unthinkable.

In nature, there is no such thing as miracles. Anything is possible as long as it coincides with her natural laws (i.e. vibration, gravity, polarity, gender [masculine and feminine], compensation, and karma, among many others). Every living thing and every force of energy abides by these laws. This is one of the big secrets of life.

The ether links itself to the human mind and is the force that connects all forms of matter, filling in every gap of space. It has blessed us with the ability to become one with nature and everything within it. Nature's power is available to humanity through the influence of thought, meaning we may produce the object within our thoughts. According to *The Master Key System*, this belief is also known as the **law of attraction**: that "the mind is creative, and will automatically correlate with its object and bring it into manifestation."[101]

There is a vibrational language that talks to this ethereal atmosphere. The human mind is static, but thought is dynamic, and its vibration is energy absorbed from the ether. If an individual possesses the power or ability to act on it, it may crystallize, which is the **law of action**.

In order to manifest the things you want in life, engage in **actions** that support your thoughts. So, a warrior may harness the power of thought internally through exercises in breathing and meditation. These practices involve the physical and mental activity of channeling energy from the inner core and connecting it to the atmosphere around us.

To gain what you want to experience in your life, visualize it in your mind and choose it with the feeling in your heart. Research in **epigenetics** from biologists such as Dr. Bruce Lipton indicates that human DNA has a *direct* effect on our physical world, and our emotions alter our DNA, which changes the world around us.[102]

It has become a common misconception that our beliefs and feelings do not affect the world outside of our bodies, which is an outrageous claim as the outside world is a reflection of the world we hold within. If there is harmony within, then there will be tranquility on the outside. If there is discord within, then there will be chaos outside.

All you have to do is open your eyes and see for yourself what most of the causes of poverty, famine, corruption, crime, murder, and war stem from. When chaos reigns in the world, it is my opinion that this is mostly due to divisions in our social, political, and religious beliefs (ego).

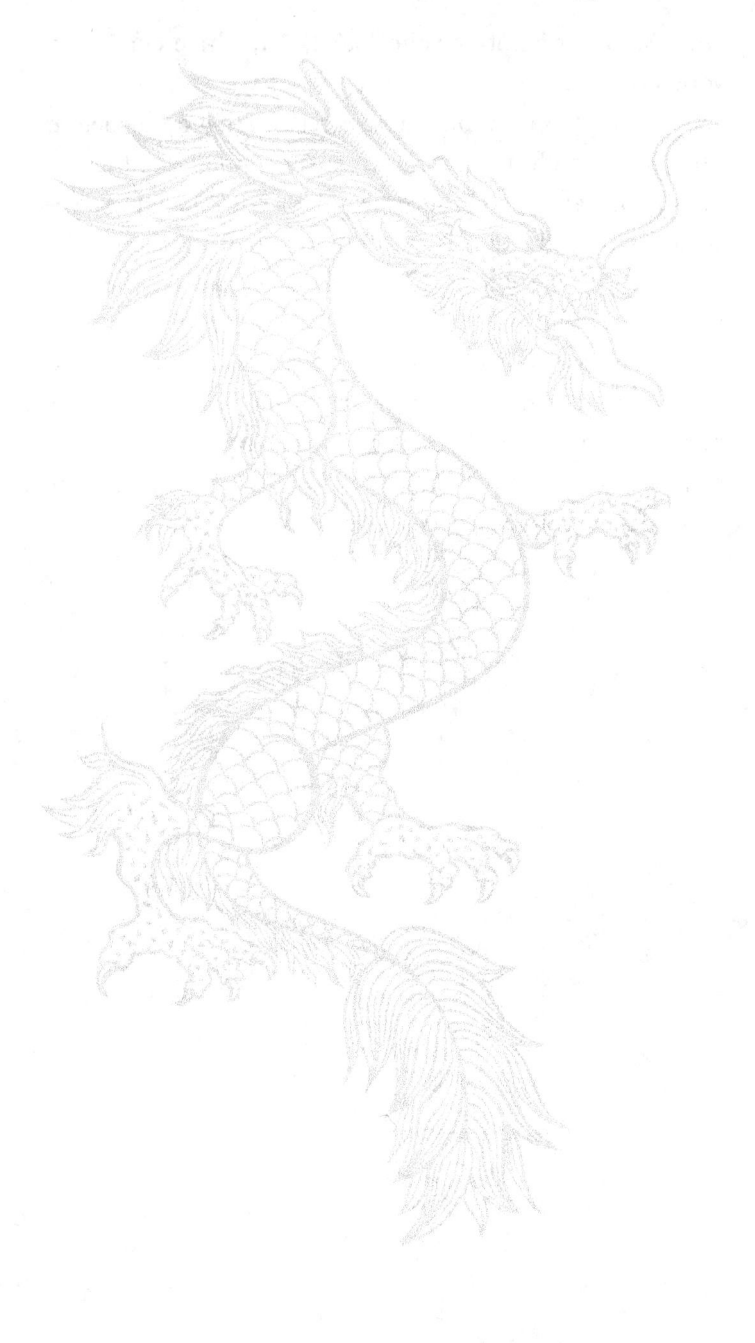

CHAPTER 11: POWER IN ALLIANCE

The second position that gives us power is the accumulated thoughts, ideas, and experiences from the **minds of man,** meaning other men and women both past and present. This is why collaboration is crucial for our advancement.

In business, it's proven that small teams, conference calls, and alignment meetings create tremendous results. I saw this while working at AT&T for fifteen years. The lessons I learned there contributed to my understanding of the essential components—not just in business, but in martial arts as well.

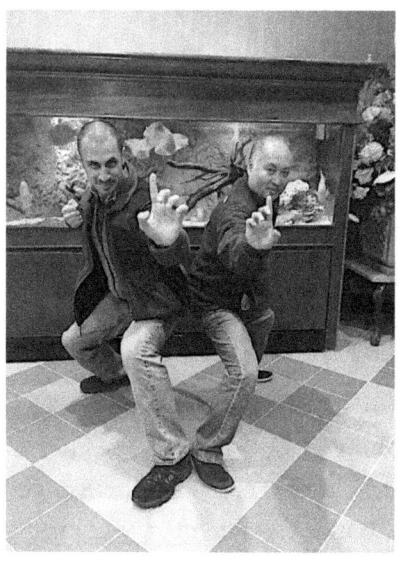

Both martial arts philosophies and applications involve inducing others to cooperate with your purpose. This is the cause for learning martial arts. You need a teacher, classmates, and opponents. These are all effects to help you learn, practice, and overcome challenges. The teacher presents the conflict, your classmates help with the struggle, and your adversaries present the challenge, all of which stimulates your growth.

Martial arts provide a consistent conflict, which a warrior requires for their development. Since martial arts apply to both the internal and external self, without a conflict in both, there can be no advancement for the individual.

If you ever feel comfortable with martial arts or think you have mastered them, this means that deep down, you think you have mastered the world. However, in reality, your ego is massive and you have a long way to go on your journey.

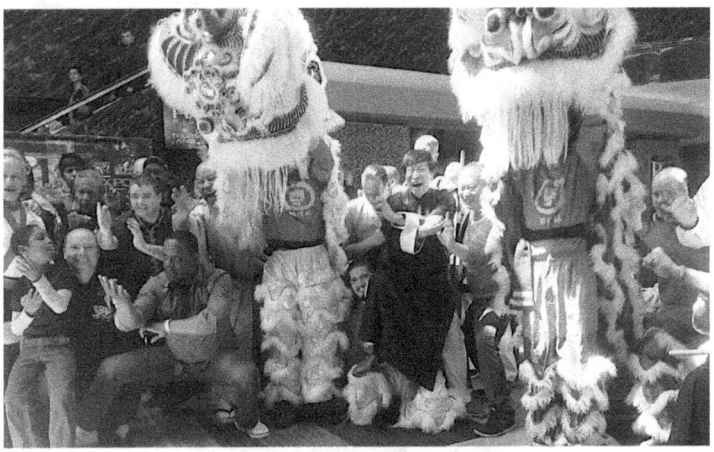

It takes an open mind and humility to enhance your consciousness, and if you are still closed tightly, then your ego is holding you back. There is no place for egotism here, because you can't do this alone. Remember, <u>you must give to receive power</u>. So, give love to your brotherhood, dismiss their faults, and serve them so they get what they want. You will get more of what you want in return.

Allow your optimism to flow freely and naturally. This way of thinking attracts positive and influential people into your life. Humility, tolerance and open-mindedness create readiness, and when you are ready, the dragon and tiger appear.

THE DRAGON AND TIGER APPEAR

Part of this chapter and the subsequent gates convey the attainment of power through the **mental** realm, the world inside, where all truth and lasting power come from. We require knowledge to possess power and we require wisdom to keep it, especially as we mature.

In the story of Bodhidharma, we saw that his creative imagination was kicked into high gear when he met the Shaolin Monks, who gave him the material to build his legacy. This story is your first lesson in attaining power from others.

No matter what and how much you know, it's best to further your knowledge through collaboration with other minds. **No man can achieve immortality alone**, and no martial artist can attain high power without the support of others. So, assemble knowledge from others and apply it through action with others, whether they are allies or enemies.

An alliance is the combination of two or more people who work together in the spirit of harmony to obtain a definite purpose. This association is why respect is an essential virtue in martial arts. It's honorable to respect both your training brothers and opponents *in the same manner*. If today's martial arts teachers don't teach their students the lessons of honor, integrity, and respect, they still have a lot to learn themselves.

All forms of cooperation implemented in the spirit of harmony are the foundation of gaining power. When martial arts techniques are carried out with mutual benefit and persistence towards the objective, then all parties involved are halfway towards their goal.

Your karma determines how far you will get with this. You may not understand it entirely, but the advantage of having power is learning from and working with others, and most importantly, with your **authentic intention.**

Power is energy, and each mind is limited in the amount of potential it can hold or emanate. However, the combination of multiple minds working *together* in harmony creates more energy and more vibration, thus power is inevitable.

The same goes for practice. The more you practice a technique and apply energy into your actions, the more your vibration and power increases, especially when combined with others. Take your techniques for example. You can practice them until you're blue in the face, but if you don't have a teacher or training partner to give you their observations and corrections, your methods may be poorly executed due to your posture, delivery, or energy placement. By yourself, you can develop good form (technique), but with the help of others, you can develop the perfect form.

Our friendships hold the secret of real power, especially when we harmoniously surround ourselves with the minds of others. The gathering of more than one mind increases the energy, creating a surge in the elevation of conductivity, which becomes part of each person in the group.

The Gracie family became legendary innovators of Brazilian jiu-jitsu and reshaped martial arts across the globe. Likewise, in the early twenty-first century, Greg Jackson's training camp housed an alliance of great champions in MMA.

In his first ten years of martial arts training, Bruce Lee was unknown and persistently worked on developing his philosophies and techniques. He didn't tap into the potential of his real power until he started collaborating with other martial artists such as James Yimm Lee, Chuck Norris, and Danny Inosanto, along with different styles such as fencing and boxing.

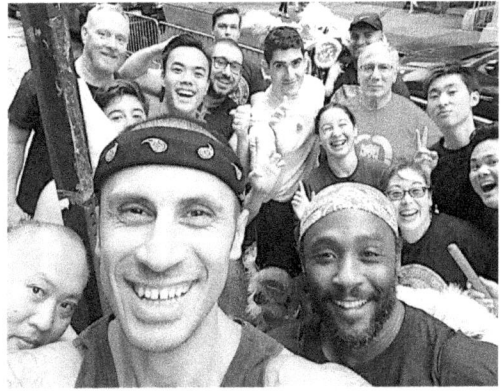

What we can learn from this is that **we all take on the nature and the habits of those we associate with**. The evidence of this is all around us. So, it's imperative to find an environment that suits your needs in obtaining your goals. Those who succeed in life are successful because of the people they learn from, practice with, or compete against—generating their power to rise above and beyond the rest.

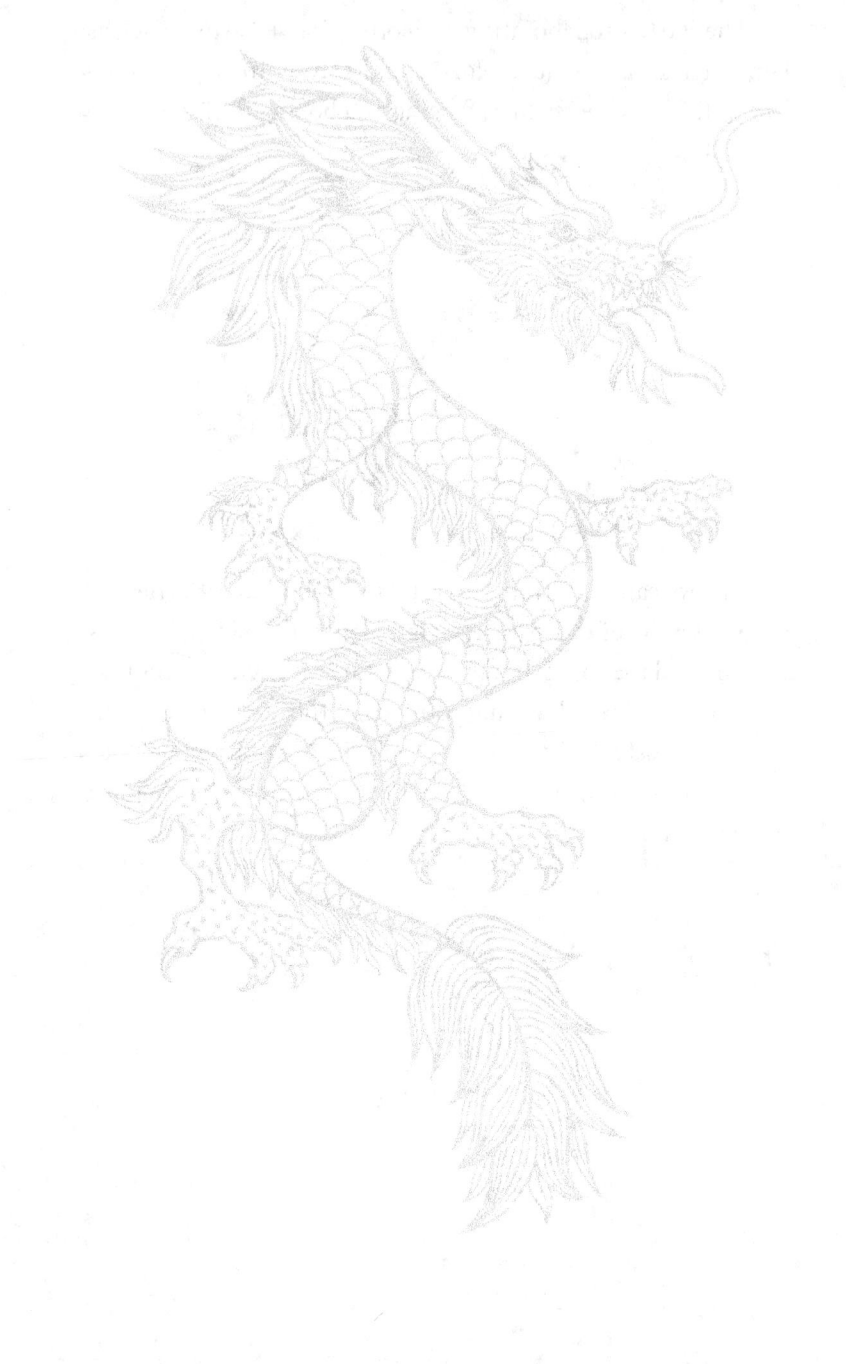

CHAPTER 12:
POWER IN PRACTICE

"You can only fight the way you practice."

— Miyamoto Musashi[103]

The third position that gives us power is **our actions** or the work we put into something. Many people believe that the physical world is the "be all and end all" of everything. Therefore, they don't understand or neglect the spiritual aspects of training altogether. Most search for power externally, overlooking the soul and its subconscious connection to the universal mind, which is the creative force of nature and everything within it.

Those like Musashi, who have reached **enlightenment,** found that they attained power when they aligned their conscious efforts with their subconscious (the universal mind). The enlightened came to understand the method and basic principles of thought transferred into action as cause produces effects.

In my opinion, most of the information today, especially on social media, is regurgitated and distributed by imitators (copycats) without a true understanding of it. For example, they may quote Buddha or something similar because it's trendy, yet have no concept of Buddhist tenets, nor have they ever read any of the sutras.

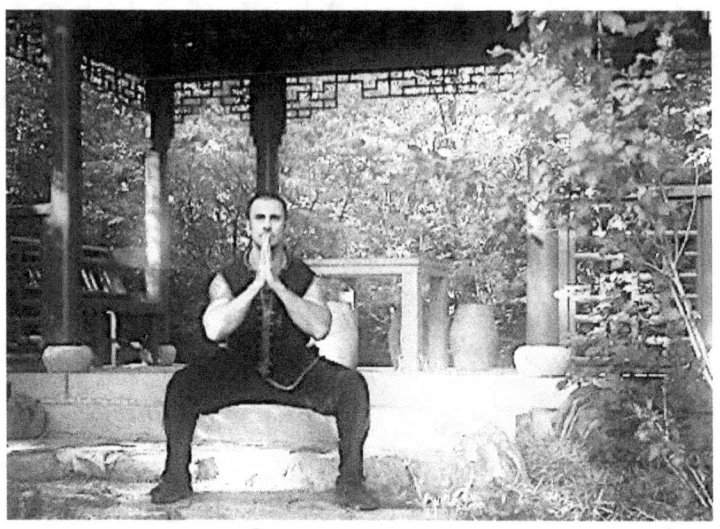

In every genre, many people are trying to obtain massive amounts of followers and get rich quickly without any real understanding or experience of what they are saying, doing, or posting, especially regarding spirituality.

No matter what anybody says or does, you have to find out the truth for yourself and experience it in order for it to be authentic. **The true knowledge and understanding of all power** (physical, mental, or spiritual), **has to be earned through practice and experience**.

KNIFE OR DEATH

In 2018, I participated in a reality show for the History Channel called *Forged In Fire: Knife or Death*. The show was an obstacle course for contestants with forged blades to cut through different objects for the quickest time, and the winner of the course would compete for a grand prize of $25,000.

For months, I trained so hard for the competition, only to lose by missing the cut of one strap on the very last obstacle. At the time, I was just grateful for the opportunity, but after I digested what had happened during filming, I realized how close I came to winning and that I made a huge mistake—I rushed through the course. I was very disappointed with myself. Honestly, it was devastating.

Before filming took place, I met one of the hosts of the show, former world wrestling champion Bill Goldberg, who gave me some encouraging advice. He said, "don't leave anything out on the course that a couple of months from now you can look back on with regret." What he said planted a seed in my subconscious mind, and I ended up doing exactly what he said. I was the only contestant on our show who did not finish the course. Within a few weeks after filming, I developed deep negative feelings and became depressed.

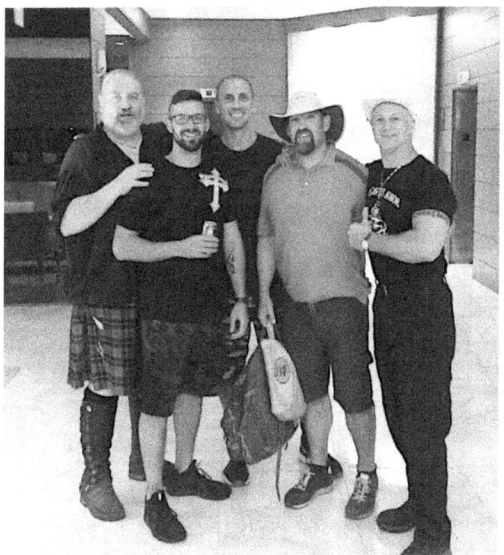

It wasn't just losing that got to me, although losing was a big part of it, especially since it would have created more opportunities for me. The overall experience of flying first class, staying in a five-star hotel, and being treated like a V.I.P. made me emotional because I felt special. I was swept away by the actor's life (ego).

As my mind became flooded with negative thoughts and emotions in the following months, I started attracting more negativity in my life, business, and relationships and eventually got cut from the show altogether, since I was the only one that didn't finish the course.

I learned a lot from that experience, but the most crucial lesson was that practicing was not enough. I needed to practice accurately to win (Musashi), not just physically but mentally and spiritually. Wielding a blade is useless without a strong mind needed to focus and the spirit of cutting through everything in life with precision. Precision requires perfect practice, which takes time, energy, and effort.

I have made my peace with the failure, which seems trivial now, made some friends (the other contestants on the show), and gained the experience of a lifetime. To live is to learn, and learning requires practice.

On your journey, stay open, humble, and receptive to both old and new information. Read helpful books. Those who pursue power often fail if they lack the proper knowledge or plans necessary for its attainment.

FARMER HARVESTING CROPS

A farmer doesn't waste time explaining to his son how to bring in the harvest when he's teaching him how to plant seeds. The process goes step by step. There is a season for planting seeds and a season for reaping the harvest, and these never happen at the same time.

Like reaping a harvest of crops, any power you seek must be earned, which takes time, energy, and effort. You will never keep your power for long unless you continue to earn it. Never forget that power must be earned, which takes time and persistent effort.

Remember chapter two, <u>nature awaits your direction</u>. It takes no effort to say, "I want this and I want that." You have to make a decision in your mind, put all of your faith towards that decision, and act on it. During the process, stay optimistic and allow constructive thoughts to permeate your mind.

Be patient, because the harvest takes time. The more time you allow, the more momentum you will gain. And the more your stimulation will intensify, your plans will take shape, and you will get a better comprehension. When you consider the positive impact that your results will have on your life and the lives of others, you will allow whatever time it takes for your power to unfold.

There is enough power in the universe to tap into and cultivate for your benefit. This knowledge enables you to live the way you want to live.

"If we are blessed with some great reward, such as fame or fortune; It's because of the fruit of a seed planted by us in the past."

— Bodhidharma[104]

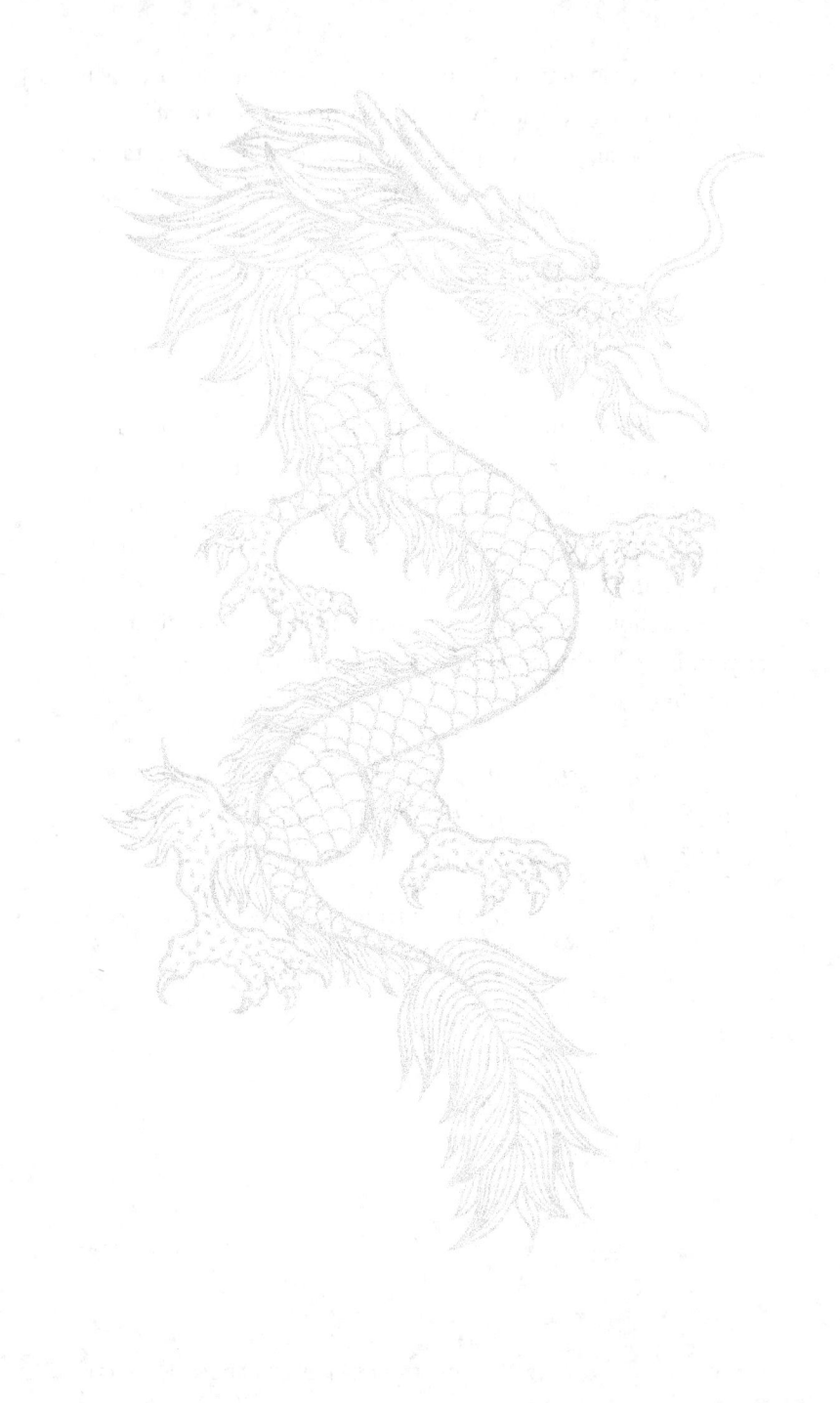

CHAPTER 13: PHYSICAL POWER

Life is most fruitful if you follow nature's law of sowing the seeds in one season and reaping the harvest in another. In the physical world, the natural laws govern the physical health of your body. If you violate those laws, your health diminishes. You can't keep the vigor of youth if you can't stay healthy, and this requires both health-consciousness and power-consciousness.

If you're addicted to and enslaved by your cell phone, social media, video games, television, pornography, over-eating, smoking cigarettes, getting drunk, or using narcotics, then your potential to generate power is limited.

In my opinion and from my experiences, you can connect both the mind and body to conquer many of the addictions, bad habits, illnesses, and concerns that pose a threat to your wellbeing.

> *"Union and conscious relation of these centers of being within us (brain and solar plexus), give us good health, strength, beauty, and youth on the physical plane, and opens the door for divine revelation to the soul."*
>
> — Dr. Julia Seton[105]

In essence, we may create a feeling of healing and develop power without the interference of negative forces from our mind. And we may generate the tremendous potential energy that we all hold within to improve our wellbeing.

This gate on the healing qualities of internal energy and the mind-body connection is specific to the attainment of physical power, and it requires discipline. A warrior who is aware of their internal energy, its strength, its feeling, and the potential for its expression becomes a **conductor of power**. The conductor keeps their strength in its place and distributes energy wisely, applying force quickly and effortlessly without thought or hesitation. The warrior eventually becomes the master, and the world becomes his servant.

THE SOLAR PLEXUS

The sun is the director of light and nature is its recipient. We all have an internal sun within our bodies called the **solar plexus**, which is the nerve center that distributes the energy our body generates. When this inner sun rises and radiates thermal energy, nature and all of those within it are the recipients of this magnificent magnetic light. The master is the conductor of this light, and many people are more than willing to follow him or her to receive it.

> *"The great creative energy of the universe is always flowing through us just as a current runs along the line, and this passing in of the finer etheric currents to be used in the rebuilding and vitalizing of the body and mind, and the passing out again from the physical body in lines of electric force, is what constitutes*

> *the human aura, and those who are actively alive in their radiation are called magnetic and attractive."*
>
> — Dr. Julia Seton[106]

When the body is radiating brilliant light, the body's structure is in proper alignment, the chest is open, and the sun is at its peak, shining brightly. The highest point of this sun hovers above a solid foundation (a strong, well-postured body), a majestic mountain if you will, creating power in any action or reaction.

This light-vitality-power that illuminates from your body is apparent because the body aligns itself to receive and distribute an abundance of energy in circulation both within the atmosphere, as well as within the body itself. The organization of the body maintains balance, and when applying any form of motion or physical action, this balance helps to cultivate your energy to properly emit the light. Our nerves discharge this light force throughout the entire body and then radiate it into the atmosphere. Those ready to receive this light will follow the leader of this magnificent sun.

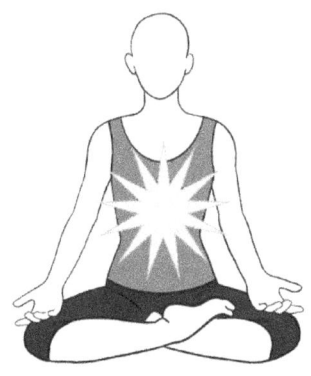

> *"The Solar Plexus has been likened to the sum of the body, because it is the central point of distribution for the energy, which the body is constantly generating. This energy is very real energy and this sun is a very real sun, and the energy is being distributed by very real nerves to all parts of the body, and is thrown off in an atmosphere, which envelopes the body."*
>
> — Charles F. Haanel[107]

ENERGY PROJECTION

In life, it's natural for people to contribute to the effects of our stresses, anxieties, pain, and closures. Although it's tempting, it's better to *not* shy away from confrontation. Instead, remain open and give your time, effort, and **positive energy** to others.
- Let your light shine.
- Let them feel your power.
- Become a source of strength and courage for them.
- Share your wisdom with them by radiating love, passion, and optimism.

This personal strength will allow your sun to shine and your body to break through all blockages that constrict your breathing and the distribution of your energy.

When you do this, there is no limit to the distance that your electrical and magnetic waves can travel, as they have tremendous force. And the force we project into the atmosphere can magnify our spiritual vibration.

When we apply the energy of emotions into our words and actions, our heart creates electrical and magnetic waves that extend from our **solar plexus** into the atmosphere around us. This magnetism is our **aura**, and these waves of energy magnify well beyond where our heart physically resides.[108] This magnification constitutes an *ethereal projection* of your energy or spiritual vibration (see diagram), since the ether field is an ocean of energy that is all around us in the atmosphere, connecting everything together.

The same goes for the transfer of **qi energy** from one human being to another. **Qi** is our vital life force, and it divides into inner and outer strength. Inner qi flows through the meridians of the body, while external qi is the circle of energy we project into the atmosphere through our thoughts, breath, emotions, and actions. When we master the mind and body, our electricity radiates outward according to our vibration.

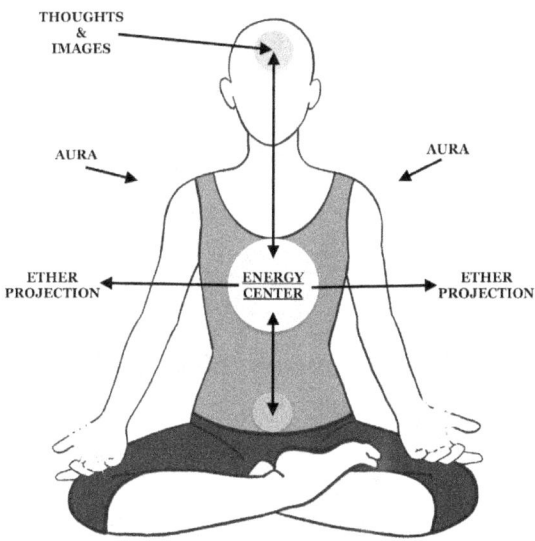

The influence of energy can project *anywhere* in nature. Wherever you are right now, this moment affects all of the space around you. Your vibration is continuously fluctuating as you read this, and the developing implications affect your overall consciousness, creating a change in the awareness of others. Some call this "the butterfly effect." Whatever it is, I believe that we are all parts of the whole, and that our actions determine our results, not just for ourselves, but for others as well.

Transferring qi energy allows an individual to heal or hurt humanity by making others stronger or weaker depending on their cause or motive. It is also worth noting that our emotions impact the distribution of our power, energy, and abilities. Therefore, any anxiety, fear, or stress can decrease momentum. These emotions can cause blockages that create headaches and nausea, jaw tension, stomach tightening, and congestion in the sinuses, throat, and chest.

As a result, it is crucial to deal with negative emotions by breathing and keeping a positive mental attitude. Things may get dark, and everything within you may want to quit, crawl into a dark hole somewhere, and completely fall apart. The way to fight darkness is with light. So, stay strong, stay positive, and stay focused. Use the breathing and meditation techniques mentioned to help fight the negative emotions you are facing and let your light shine.

LIFE FORCE

The human body has 108 **pressure points** consisting of a multitude of currents. The electricity within the human body is called *qi* (pronounced chee) in Chinese, *ki* (pronounced key) in Japanese, and *prana* (pronounced pra-na) in Hindi.

This life force is the body's version of ethereal power that results in the combination of breath, blood, and electricity. In essence, qi is what powers the strength of the body, the force of the mind, and the energy of the spirit. We cultivate it by practicing martial arts, yoga, and meditation, and can be interpreted in a variety of ways:

1. BREATH: Connecting your mind and body to the ether, by breathing in the air. Life begins with the way we breathe, use our respiration, and circulate oxygen throughout the body. All power in the body requires active breath control. By controlling the air pressure, you can direct the distribution of qi throughout the body. This means inflating and deflating the body's air pressure by breathing in, holding, and releasing the breath slowly for different lengths of time, as well as the force of air used to reach the internal organs and the depths of your inner core.
2. ELECTRICITY: The human body is a sphere of energy, and within it there are many smaller circles responsible for the cultivation and movement of potential electrical power. As this power flows, it becomes kinetic energy. When it vibrates at an increasingly rapid speed, it turns into thermal energy. Then the body emits tremendous heat.
3. FORCE: As in raising your vibration, increasing your forward motion or movement in pursuit of something, or gaining of momentum during your actions. The faster the rate of penetration (breaking through barriers) or vibration, the more heat is generated, which pumps blood through the veins. This friction strengthens the mind and increases the spirit to perform the activity.

In the Shaolin and Taoist kung fu systems, qigong, acupuncture, and traditional Chinese medicine, qi is a common term. It is the energy that resonates in all living things and is the electro-current that transmits through your body.

Qi is electricity, similar to the force of **electromagnetism** within the earth. It is all-powerful and always present and needs to be harnessed and cultivated through the proper channels of the body.

THE CINNABAR FIELD

There are meridians in the body that circulate this electricity (qi), and they are connected by 108 pressure points (pressure valves). These meridians all relate to specific glands and internal organs.

Everything within the body bands together, and seven main energy hubs known as *chakras* (Hindi) run along the centerline of the body. In ancient Chinese practices, these centers are broken down into the three chambers called *daantins* (Cantonese).

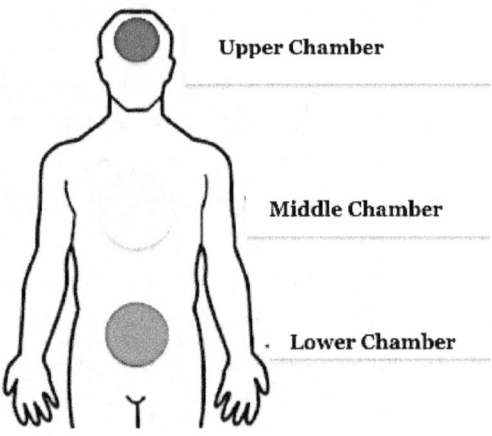

The electro-current flows throughout the body, and up and down the chakras or daantins. When unobstructed, they generate the momentum of power within you. When connected with the mind, the body can coordinate movements to produce a high-quality flow of breath, blood, and electricity. This in turn allows the body and mind's intention to simultaneously move with great force.

The vast storehouse of potential electrical energy within the body resides in the lower pit of the abdomen referred to as the lower daantin, otherwise known as the "cinnabar field." There are three daantin fields, and each is associated with a particular color. The lower chamber is red and labeled "the root of life." The middle chamber is yellow, consisting of the solar plexus and the heart. Finally, the upper chamber is blue, and sits at the crown of the head, as the home of the brain and the pineal gland.

The abdomen is a region of extraordinary power and the source of qi energy in the body. The inner chamber is where qi is harnessed and cultivated for ascent to the solar plexus for distribution throughout the body and into the atmosphere. In other words, the cinnabar field is where the sun rises and the solar plexus is the solar noon.

The lower daantin cultivates energy and is the force responsible for creating life; creation is one of the highest forms of power in the universe. This power comes from within and can cure everything in your life if you learn to harness its energy and use it for your benefit. However, having a capability like this does not come quickly; it takes years of practice and mastery of meditation to perfect.

The kung fu system of *Hung Ga Kuen* (Hung Family Fist) has many daantin-cultivating exercises within all of its forms. Most kung fu styles do. These methods make the style complete for both internal and external factors. It utilizes internal breathing for external application, a vital element missing from many other martial art styles.

Whenever we harness this electricity, its healing effects remove all blockages within the body and this increases our power. The stronger your circulation, the healthier you become. As a result, injuries heal faster, your skin may become smoother, your eyes brighter and sharper, and your lungs free and clear.

As energy becomes thermal and reaches every part of your body, you can experience the feelings and sensations of electricity pulsating throughout your extremities. Furthermore, when the energy flows to the **pineal chakra** in the head, you may feel a relaxed, cool-blue euphoria.

As the power streams through the upper body to the arms, you may feel a vivacity that shoots out through your fingertips. When the force resonates in your inner core, calmness and stability progresses down to the roots of your body (the legs) and descends to the bottoms of your feet. In this sense, **a human being is like a tree and is an extension of the earth**.

THE ELECTROMAGNETIC FIELD

Just as humans have a cinnabar field in the abdomen, which is a special place of power, our earth has a **nucleus of energy** as well. The ground below us has a dynamic source of electromagnetism, which is a variation of the potential electric energy we carry within our bodies.

Electromagnetism is essential to the motion of electricity in human beings. Our planet offers unlimited amounts of electromagnetic energy that can be harnessed by anyone to magnify their qi. This concept applies to the ether as well.

The earth has meridians similar to the body that course within it and connects all the special places of power. These meridians in the ground are called "dragon paths" in the East, and "ley lines" in the West. All over the world, there are sacred temples and pyramids built on these electromagnetic locations by occultists who sought to harness their energy for power. There are also places where you may feel whole or rejuvenated. These locations have high levels of electromagnetic energy—you may not see them, but they are there.

According to many practitioners of traditional Chinese medicine, human beings are progressively losing their connection to this electromagnetic energy, especially in the last century due to the increase in technology. Therefore, be mindful of how we treat the planet and our bodies to harness this energy to its full capacity.

As a result of technology, life can move very fast. But when you learn to slow down your mind and avoid distractions, then your potential energy and the electromagnetic energy of the earth can kinetically join. This is why it's crucial to stay present in every moment and slow life down to make the most of it. Taking a time out to meditate in nature is the best way to harness and cultivate your inner strengths.

When a warrior needs to increase their energy for more power, there are many ways to do so. For example, you may draw strength from nutrition, exercise, meditation, or the earth by placing your left hand[¶¶¶] on a tree or removing your shoes on grass (grounding). The first time I tried this I thought it was eccentric, but I could actually feel the energy transferring into my body through my hands and feet as if they were electricity conductors.

Many people don't realize that natural energy can be drained or restored; however, just by maintaining an open mind, these concepts will further your understanding of life. Energy transfers can occur between nature and other people, yet our divorce from nature and lack of meditation prevents us from ascending, because we have closed the gates to the higher power within us.

¶¶¶ According to Hindi beliefs, the left hand receives energy and the right hand sends it out.

The human body is at its best when its kinetic energy is flowing freely and naturally. This is why we eat clean, warm-up, stretch, and practice breathing techniques in martial arts, as it removes all blockages in the body to generate the best results for training.

ENERGY WORK

Qigong is the ultimate form of practice to maintain physical health, heal the body, increase vitality, find peace of mind, and connect to the spirit. These potential energy development exercises preserve the body through the following:

1. Injury prevention and recovery
2. Internal conditioning
3. Maintaining overall health and wellness

The primary focus is to harness and cultivate qi and move it throughout the body. We can accomplish this method of enhancing energy kinetically when the blood, breath, and electricity move freely without any blockages.

Many qigong methods are used internally to invigorate the organs, but they are also known to:

- Reduce mental stress.
- Revitalize the body.
- Strengthen the immune system.
- Enhance the body's nervous, circulatory, cardiovascular, respiratory, lymphatic, digestive, urinary, and reproductive systems.

When bone marrow shrinks or dies, the body's immune system and cell reproduction diminish. Qi energy revitalizes your internal strength by expanding your body's energy fields and this is why qigong is important.

In the past, many people believed that qigong was a form of black magic due to its healing properties and results that appeared to be miracles. Moreover, when these practices weren't executed correctly, they tended to hurt others instead of healing them. Thus, these malpractices led to mysticism and fear.

In modern times, especially in new age mixed martial arts, most practitioners dismiss the existence of qi energy or have become wary of its practices. This is due to deceitful masters and their outrageous claims of discharging orbs of energy from their palms. These false claims are dishonorable and defy the laws of nature, which results in bad karma. Unfortunately, as a result, kung fu and karate have inherited poor reputations from those with rigid ideas and preconceived notions that all qi exercises are nonsense.

Fortunately, qigong has become more widespread and accepted as a form of therapeutic healing and part of martial arts training. The gift of healing is compelling, especially as most traditional Chinese medicine practices can decrease pain, stress, sickness, disease, some cancers, and paralysis by harnessing thermal energy and transferring heat to restore the body to a neutral state. These methods require mental focus and specific breathing techniques to cultivate energy by elevating the body's temperature. This way, thermal energy can move wherever it's needed to rehabilitate the body or part of it.

Author's note: *When I fractured my rib in jiu-jitsu class, jiu-jitsu did not have any internal breathing exercises to help with the healing. The kung fu exercises of qigong were one of the major components of my speedy recovery. In just three weeks, I was back on the mat.*

IRON WIRE

Usually regarded as family practice, qigong has been passed down from generation to generation. There are many different forms and styles of qigong, but initially meditative and combative qigong were used by Buddhist and Taoist monks for centuries to achieve immortality and were withheld from the mainstream because the monks were isolated by temple life.

In the era of the southern Shaolin Temple, the monks combined meditative qigong breathing methods with the five animals fighting system to develop a potent training regimen for both health and combat. The monks found these breathing exercises beneficial for the circulation of breath, blood, and electricity. They magnified their breathing to inflate and deflate the body's air pressure, and strenuously exerted constant tension in the muscles of their extremities. This strengthened their muscle tissue, bones, organs, tendons, and ligaments.

These techniques cultivated and increased the power of the mind-body connection. When you're hurt or in pain, thermal energy must reach the injured body part to heal it. As qi energy can sometimes get stuck in certain areas, it must be released and moved to the rest of the body for circulation. The meridians join arteries and nerves that are responsible for blood flow, and when the blood circulates efficiently, the body is healthy.

One particular form (kata) that creates tremendous power is the "iron wire." The iron wire increases energy and improves oxygen and blood circulation. As a result, the weak can become stronger, conquer illnesses, and live long and healthy lives.

The iron wire belongs to schools of "hard style" kung fu, which originated in the Southern Shaolin Temple. Revered as one of the last treasures of Shaolin, the iron wire was almost lost to humanity forever. Thankfully, the monks who escaped the destroyed temple dispersed the Shaolin secrets.

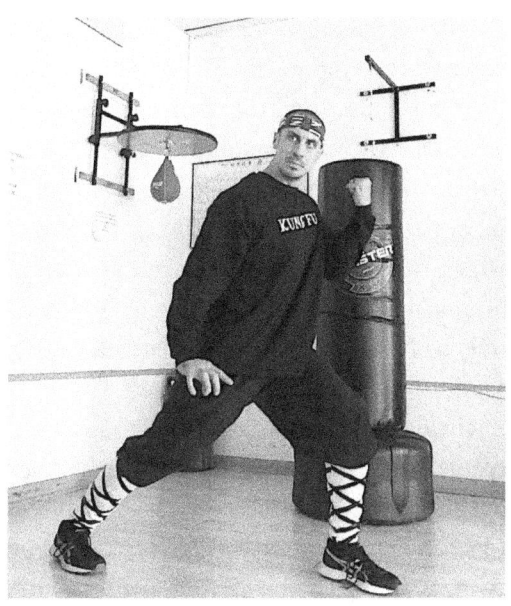

The iron wire fist,**** known in Cantonese as *tid sin kuen*, was cultivated and perfected by a great master named Leung Gwan (1813-1886), who went by the nickname Tid Kiu Sam ("Iron Bridge III").

Tid Kiu Sam was initially known as one of the "Ten Tigers of Kwangtung," who were known as the greatest fighters in southern China at the time. Tid Kiu Sam was a favorite disciple of a great warrior monk from the southern Shaolin Temple named Gwok Yan. Gwok Yan was famous for his mastery of the martial arts and having no rivals equal to him. The iron wire form that Tid Kiu Sam learned from Gwok Yan was dominant and made him very strong.

During his travels, Tid Kiu Sam came across a convent of nuns, where an extraordinary master and head nun, Yun Shen, resided.

**** This short biography is an excerpt taken from the book *Iron Thread* (1932) by author and legendary martial artist Lam Sai Wing.

She had links to the Southern Shaolin Temple and allowed him to stay at her convent temporarily. Through Buddhist tradition, she offered her hospitality and they gained each other's respect, so Yun Shen shared the missing links to complete the iron wire form, known as the "twitter of the dragon."

Tid Kiu Sam was already dynamic, but the missing pieces gained through this alliance made him even better. After completing and mastering the iron wire form, Tid Kiu Sam displayed immense power and became a legend, whose skill was unsurpassed.[109]

The iron wire form was passed on from Tid Kiu Sam to a select few and became exclusive to an inner circle of his kung fu lineage (Hung Ga Kuen). The exercise gained notoriety and became more widespread when demonstrated by Chinese folk hero Wong Fei Hung (1847-1925), who passed it on to a broader audience of the Hung family. Unfortunately, it appears that through the centuries, the form has been changed or watered down, and because of this, there are so many different versions claiming to be the original. Regardless of which version you practice, the iron wire is exclusive and still regarded as a treasure. This unique training method is revered by most Hung Kuen practitioners and not easily given away.

However, due to the comforts of technology, there are no secrets any longer and the iron wire form is shown on social media sites such as YouTube and the sequence is also detailed in some books. If you do not have access to a hands-on Sifu to teach you the Hung Kuen version of Iron Wire, I recommend the YouTube videos from Sifu Ng Ping Kuen or Sifu Lam Chun Fai, who both have over half a century of experience with the form. Use these videos in conjunction with Lam Sai Wing's book, *Iron Thread* (1932).

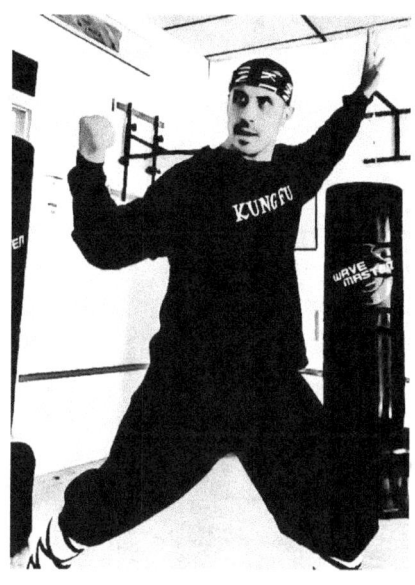

Without guidance or a solid kung fu foundation, the concepts will be difficult to grasp for some beginners and useless if not performed correctly, so I highly recommend hiring a teacher. If you practice grappling arts like judo or jiu-jitsu, you will recognize some of the postures in the form that represent lapel grabs (grips), hand locks, low horse stance, throws, and chokes (cross collar, Ezequiel, bow & arrow, and others).

Note: I have been practicing this form almost every day for the last several years for the sole purpose of learning and understanding the concepts, as well as increasing my physical strength and acquiring robust health. As time passed, the form changed, and so have I. Every time I practice, I learn something new about myself and I feel something different. I practice in solitude because it helps me focus; I can pay attention to every detail, understand what my body is doing, what my mind is thinking, and what my solar plexus is feeling. Here are some key points that I have observed:

1. Go slowly, there is no need to rush this form. It should last around fifteen minutes.
2. Breathing correctly is crucial. When you perform the postures slowly and breathe in conjunction with each posture, your brain (upper chamber), solar plexus (middle chamber), and lower daantin (lower chamber) can connect.
3. When your fists are clenched, perform the moves as if you are actually holding an iron wire. Build and hold the tension in your arms from the hands to the forearms, biceps, triceps, and then shoulders. Also, keep your core tight. Only let go of the tension when you perform the posture called "twitter of the dragon."
4. I have seen this form performed thousands of times (literally), and every performer does it differently and exerts different sounds during the applications. Since kung fu can be cultish at times, everyone will swear that his or her iron wire form is the original. Then I pose the question, why is everyone's form different? In my opinion, the particular sounds needed for exertion are trivial. However, the exertion of breathing and sound is still crucial and must be utilized. Practice and try your best, which is all you can do.
5. I am a very intense individual, and when I practice, I sometimes obsess and overtrain, and I will honestly tell you that you can injure yourself while overtraining this form. I developed a sprained MCL, strained bicep tendon, as well as golfers and tennis elbow. Therefore, I advise you to take it easy and stop if you feel pain. Allow your body a couple of days to rest and recover. On the other hand, the iron wire has also helped me recover from injuries too.

If performed correctly, you will feel the effects of all three chambers (daantins) as the electrical force runs through your body. When you finish, there will be times when you feel happy, relaxed, euphoric, somber, angry, and even aggressive.

The feelings are connected to your solar plexus and I strongly believe that the energy you feel may enhance your current mood. As a result, after practice, allow about an hour to be alone so that your energy does not mix with any other. During this one-hour period:
- Don't spit.
- Don't go to the bathroom.
- Don't eat anything.
- Don't drink anything.
- Try to avoid people if you can.
- Just keep breathing until your body returns to its usual state.
- Try to avoid using any technology.

TECHNOLOGY KILLS QI

According to author and qigong master Jwing-Ming Yang, there are many distractions such as technology that prevent people from remaining focused long enough to learn and achieve mastery of their body. Many of these distractions, including cell phones, kill the generation and movement of qi energy through the body.[110] This form of technology is a type of slavery and a detriment to our physical and mental wellbeing.

As well as cell phones, there is a continuous emission of radio waves, microwaves, satellite frequencies, tower radiation, Wi-Fi, and other electronic transmissions that bombard the body regularly, and these affect our ability to produce, harness, and circulate qi effectively.

According to author Kevin Trudeau, these frequencies can cause chaos within us, and can be eliminated or at least neutralized by electromagnetic field chaos eliminators, which are pendants or devices that neutralize the electronic frequencies around you.[111]

If this chaos runs rampant, it has the potential to affect our ability to transmit and receive frequencies to the brain and limits the distribution of qi energy in the body. When you can neutralize these transmissions, your body finds balance and all of its powers can flow freely and naturally in a healthy vibrational state. Then the light from your solar plexus can shine brightly, establishing an unobstructed connection through the ether to a higher power.

CHAPTER 14: MENTAL POWER

The ancient masters of Shaolin recognized that **breathing** is the key to mastering the mind, the body, and the world. Your breath is life and an expression of your spirit. Without respiration, there is no life; there is nothing left. Our respiration is the connecting link that brings the finite and the infinite closer together.

Providence is the force that connects to our subconscious minds. This connection exists whether you call it the Great Spirit, God, Allah, Christ, Buddha, Jehovah, or Yahweh. No matter what you call it, this creative force is based on the supreme intelligence that is the one life.

I have come to the conclusion that human beings are part of that supreme intelligence. The gift of breathing comes to us directly from this creative force. So, trust in your own link, as it will help you develop faith and confidence in yourself, and it will create clarity and depth of vision to become the creator of your own destiny and a receiver of mental power.

BLACK DRAGON SWINGS ITS TAIL

Most martial artists spend the first part of their career obsessed with the physical side of training and competition. Yet, as they mature in their craft, the obsession often switches to the mental aspects, such as breathing, meditating, intuition, and feeling. These are all elements related to the **subconscious**, which we unfold in the world within.

The key to internal harmony is to unify the mind and body. For that reason, exercises such as **qigong breathing** help us to focus on connecting our breath with our mind. Qigong breathing also helps you channel the movement of qi energy. When you master your breathing, your thoughts become clearer, your physical strength increases, and your training improves dramatically.

During these breathing exercises, you can relax the mind by focusing your thoughts internally, then projecting them outwards. This harmonious alliance enables the proper distribution of power, which is dispersed through breathing while performing a technique or meditating. It's beneficial if the motion of your body connects to your breathing *simultaneously* during any action. Inhale to gather this force, then exhale to release it.

As your qigong practice matures, it will become easier to feel your energy increasing. When you finally reach the stage where you can maximize your true potential, then you can practice when conscious, have sex and enjoy it, revel in your work, and appreciate life. Everything in your existence will be enhanced because your body and mind are connected. This connection elevates your spirituality, which amplifies your martiality.[††††] When we unify our mind and body, our internal energy force moves through the body with infinite effectiveness.

To prepare your body for practice, release anything sinus-related. Eliminate internal waste such as phlegm, urine, and bowel movements from the body before exercise and meditation to avoid distraction or the circulation of poor-quality qi. However, when practicing, it's better to swallow your spit because not only does spitting dehydrate you, it releases your energy.

Particular breathing exercises such as iron wire qigong are vital because it helps with the realignment of our internal energy. It increases our lifespan by promoting the flow of qi into different

---
†††† The essence or nature of being martial with regard to martial arts.

parts of the body that need care and attention. We all have weak areas, but one of the primary focal points of this exercise is removing all blockages in the body that prevent oxygen and blood circulation.

I recognize how difficult this will be for beginners because it was for me. I strongly advise you to try this slowly at first, especially for the first few weeks. If you keep practicing this exercise, then you will be on a road to a higher level of power.

With regard to meditative breathing exercises, sometimes simple breathing is not enough, and we must reach the lower cinnabar field by force through a "corkscrew" method, learned in the iron wire form, which returns scattered qi back to the abdomen. The corkscrew method works by pushing the breath down the stomach in a circular manner, similar to the way ice cream comes out of the machine into a cone.

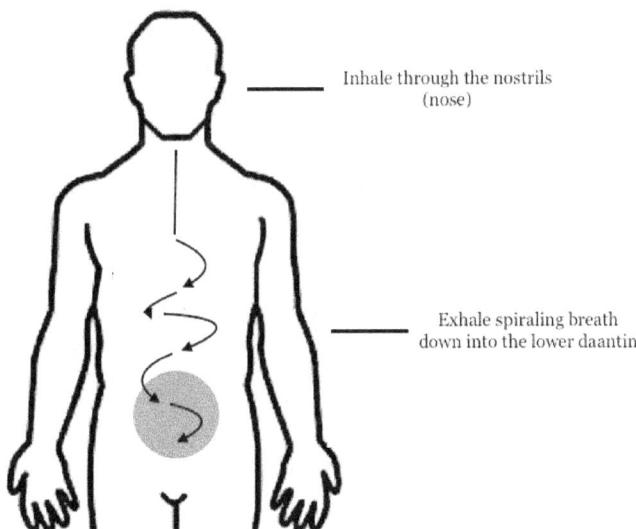

Inhale through the nostrils (nose)

Exhale spiraling breath down into the lower daantin

You may not grasp these techniques straight away and that's alright. The more you read and practice, the better your understanding will be, the more your plan will take shape, your momentum build, and your inspiration grow. In the process, your subconscious mind absorbs everything. The subconscious mind eventually gives you the power needed for discovery, development, and distribution.

Qi responds to our thoughts, actions, emotions, senses, and food. Through proper nutrition, exercising, sleeping, and practicing meditation, our breathing nourishes, manages, and circulates qi energy by breaking through obstructions in various parts of the body.

There are many times in life when the body falls out of balance or alignment, for example, sitting all day, insomnia, injury, illness, stress, junk food, sex, weather changes, body temperature fluctuations, music, or technology such as television, radios, laptops (Wi-Fi), or cell phones.

If there is a stubborn blockage, you can remove it with acupuncture, which is an excellent practice to bring the body back into realignment. Unfortunately, due to the loose translations of Cantonese and Mandarin, most Western practitioners study watered-down renditions of the art.

Therefore, find a quality practitioner who has the knowledge, experience, and reputation and stay consistent to gain the best results. You may have to test a few practitioners out before you find one who suits your needs. The important factor is how you feel afterwards—if they did their job correctly then you will feel better.

SURRENDERING TO NOW

Another important factor in gaining mental power is **staying present in the moment**. In the Zen tradition, this is one of the keys to a Shaolin monk's way of life.

When the temple bells rang, it induced total conscious presence. No matter what the monks were doing at the time, whether it was chores, practice, or meditation, the bells were so loud that the vibrations sent shockwaves to the electrical force in the monk's bodies and brought them back to a conscious presence. They were all parts of the whole, and in that moment, they recognized it. Most of the time, we don't hear the bell, and so we get lost in our stubborn thoughts, emotions, and selfishness or tasks and duties.

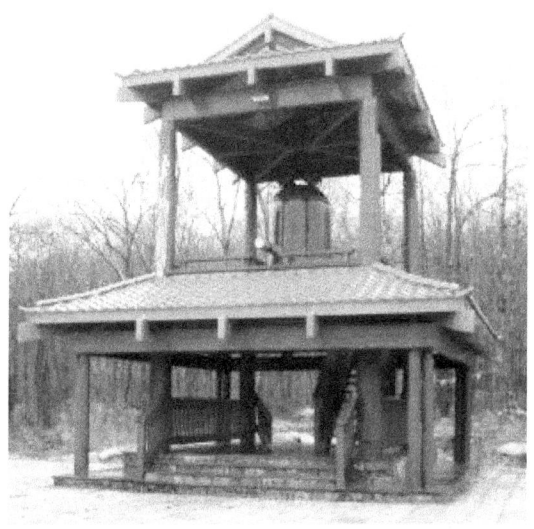

Staying present in the moment and keeping your chest open helps you breathe properly and absorb so much more of life and all of its different energies. A sedentary lifestyle, daily stress, and the overuse of technology tend to bring about blockages in the body through a lack of breathing and isolation. This obstructs the spiritual cord of the chakras, especially the force emanating from your solar plexus, which is the nerve center where your energy links to everything in nature.

When you have mental and physical awareness, breathing down the front of your open body allows qi to flow to and from the cinnabar field, and this may improve your power. Please take a moment to stand up, open your chest, inhale deeply, and exhale slowly. Do this three times and feel the energy of your breath, then sit down and continue to breathe as you read. The power of qi is generated within you, so accept it and embrace it. You have to be open and receptive for it to work.

ACTIVE POWER-CONSCIOUSNESS

An individual with power-consciousness understands nature and her laws of cause and effect, supply and demand, and increasing returns. These laws are all based on **karma** for our choices and actions in life. When we possess power-consciousness, our mind knows there is an infinite supply of energy and power within us. In nature, there is no lack or limitation—only abundance and compensation.

It's true that life is sometimes unpredictable. However, for the most part, if a master experiences problems, obstacles, or an insufficient supply to meet their needs, then deep down, they know they are the cause of the problem. For example:

- In friendships or family relationships, you choose the type of friend or family member you are, which may be fun, strong, happy, caring, giving, listening, supportive, and unselfish.
- In relationships, you choose the type of lover you are, which may be romantic and compromising. If there is no compromise from the other party, then you choose whether or not to stay in the negative relationship.
- In school, you choose the type of student you are by listening, studying, working hard, and striving to get better grades or promoted.

- In business, you choose the quality and quantity of service you provide, how attractive it is to the consumer, and your effort in providing that service in a way that makes you successful.
- In finance, you choose how to save and manage your money, the type of job you have and how well you perform it, the type of home you live in and its location, and the kind of car you drive and its condition.
- In health, you choose what you put into your body and how often you eat, sleep, read, exercise, and rest.
- In martial arts, you choose how hard you practice and whether you constantly strive for better results. If you train too hard and the results don't follow, then you choose whether or not to stay with that martial art.

Whatever you do, please pay attention to the details because thorough preparation and experience are the contributing factors that bring maximum results. A master pays attention to the details. Anyone who dwells on this higher level of consciousness, regardless of their status (whether they are considered a master or not), possesses the ability to see all their plans of action through to their end result. They demand the most out of their pursuits and endeavors, and acquire the best of everything in return for their efforts.

Moreover, when someone has the desire and persistence to see their desire through to completion, it helps them recognize all of their shortcomings or mistakes that are bringing them negative results, and in turn, take the necessary steps to correct them.

Those who have the wisdom to focus on the *cause* of the problem can make the mental corrections needed to conquer it, like everything else in life. There is no point in complaining because everything is an effect and all results are under your control.

Power-consciousness is everyone's birthright, and if it's active, the master experiences no less than what they deserve, takes full responsibility for all actions, and holds themselves accountable for any missteps. There is no such thing as blame, lack, or limitation. There are only plateaus, and you must have the mental fortitude to rise above and beyond them. The grit needed for this is called **active power-consciousness**.

A powerful mind thinks powerful thoughts. A warrior of this magnitude is an impressive listener and a dynamic speaker. They focus on attracting abundance and better conditions, and they magnify their current strengths into more power. The owner of such forces draws success into every aspect of their life. They are successful, if not at the present moment, then soon.

Power is mental security and gives a master the vitality to permeate space, among other things. This form of dynamic expansion is one of the qualities of a dragon that commands attention and magnetizes energy from others. Such people are lively, poised when they need to be, and hyper aware of their surroundings.

In any situation, <u>the entire body must be open and engaged</u>. This awareness allows a master to sense and pick up clues and intentions from associates and acquaintances. Also, this openness enables you to receive messages from nature or intuition from the subconscious mind.

The formula to discover and develop the mental strength for active power-consciousness is this: <u>meditate</u>. Use your power of visualization in meditation. This is a great strength that we possess. See, feel, and believe yourself to already be doing or possessing what you are visualizing for your life. If your goal is love, happiness, health, wealth, or power, then see the vision and then make your decisions with clarity and focus towards this goal.

Calm your heart and mind and move forward within, because that is where the connection to the infinite resides. It's buried deep within your inner core, cultivated through persistent practice in the same way as physical power is secured through exercise. This way, you may tap into it and harness the energy that creates it, which is the source of all power.

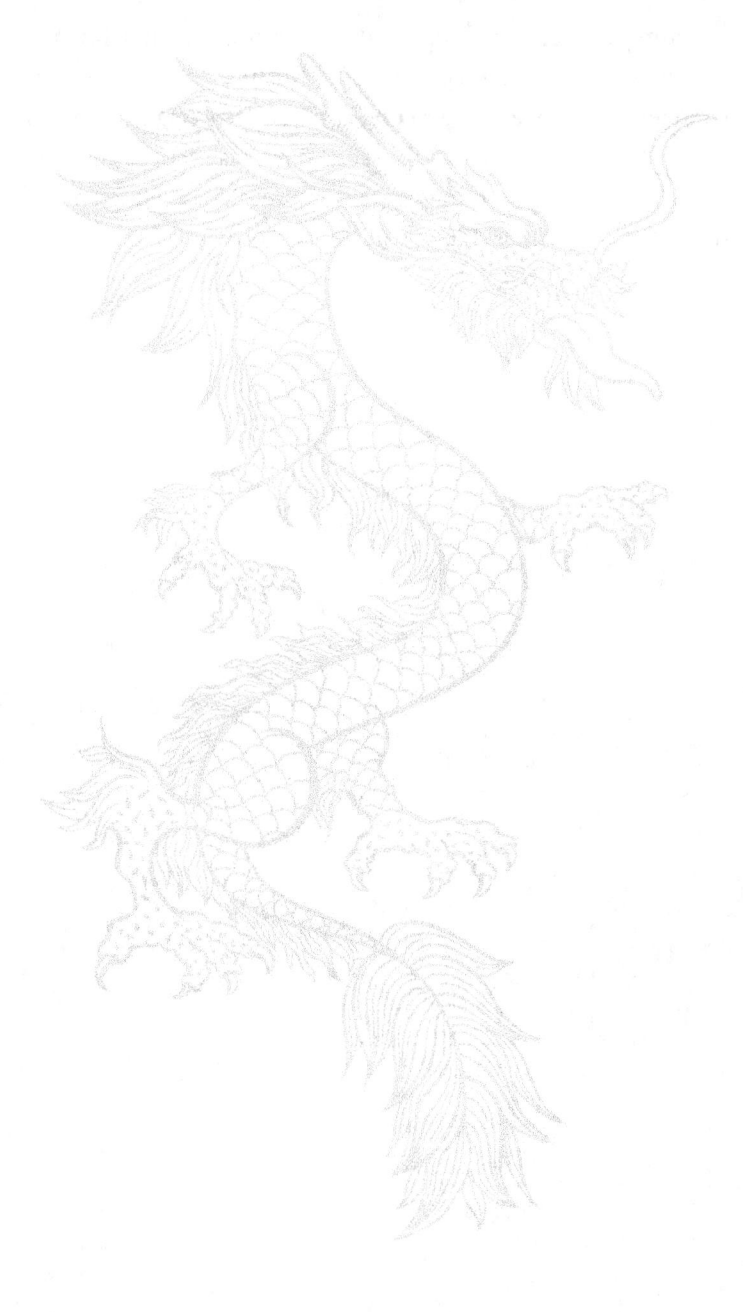

CHAPTER 15: SPIRITUAL POWER

A radio transmits frequencies from the atmosphere into sound so we can hear it. The frequency broadcasts anything from news to music. For the radio to transmit a communication, it needs energy and power. The electrical current required for the receiver to function is all around us; however, harnessing and directing the electricity is necessary. When the radio's cord is plugged into an electrical socket, the energy flows and the receiver becomes operative. The more power a radio has, the better the transmission, and the wider the range of channels it can broadcast.

Now, let's take that same concept and apply it to a human being. The human body is a shell, just like a radio, and the soul is a form of spiritual energy that is absolute. The soul is the vim and vigor that drives the human body. It is the power that connects you to everything tangible and intangible in the atmosphere.

The soul is the proverbial "cord" that runs through the body, and if it's "unplugged," then conductivity ceases to flow. As a result, energy must stream in connection with this cord. When you're open and receptive, you are in tune with the transmitter; you become the receiver and are fully accessible. This means you have spiritual awareness, called **super-consciousness**. You can practice increasing your energy flow, so that you can harness more of it from other sources.

When the soul connects to Providence, we are linked to everything in existence. This association ensures that all gates are open and all channels are free and clear to receive the full transmission of spiritual power. The spirit of Providence is where we draw our energy and power.

By contrast, having no soul means having no real power, no life, no vibration, and no energy force. This is evident when a human being dies. The body is no longer flowing with energy, so it is dead. As long as your soul is in conscious communion with the body, then you are alive.

If the soul no longer lives in the body, then it resides in the atmosphere, because energy is neither created nor destroyed. If this doesn't make sense right now, don't worry, as it will eventually.

SUPER-CONSCIOUSNESS

"You are not a human being having a spiritual experience, you are a spiritual being having a human experience."

— Pierre Teilhard De Chardin[112]

In this philosophy, power-consciousness (i.e. the mind-body connection) will not only help you in martial arts, but also in life. Now, we have established that, *where do we go from here*?

Since you are a spiritual being, your cause, unknowingly, is to obtain the principles of **super-consciousness**, which is the highest level of spirituality. In essence, super-consciousness is the motive for your soul and a topic I will explore in depth in a future publication in this series; however, I will briefly touch on it here.

You are the cause and the forces, people, and circumstances you face and experience in the external world are the effects.

To obtain super-consciousness, you have to live your life with absolute freedom. It's a spiritual sickness to live in fear under the enslavement of others and their boundaries, or under the influence of contrary or limiting thoughts and beliefs. You always have the power to dictate how far you go, how high you soar, and how long it takes to get there.

I lived the beginning of my life like a sleepwalker, and it wasn't until I started applying power in my actions that I became successful in obtaining spiritual freedom. It's one thing to read about it, another to think about it, and an entirely different thing to apply it in your everyday life and experience it for yourself.

I have always been an underdog, continually trying to better myself and improve my life. As a result, I attracted everything that mirrored the thoughts and beliefs I held within me until now. Please don't get me wrong, my life has been full of ups and downs; however, I have the ability to accept life as a rollercoaster and understand the natural laws that allow us to live spiritually, freely, and naturally. This has kept me strong and full of faith.

I may not know you personally, but I support you and wrote this for you. Right here and right now, we are changing, you and I. As a result, we are reshaping the world together for the freedom of obtaining power for mutual benefit.

The eternal laws of nature will provide the aptitude you need to obtain super-consciousness. The most basic of these laws and probably most important is the **law of vibration**, which means that everything is constantly moving and change is inevitable. Right now, you are moving forward, learning, developing, and growing. The more you apply these principles, the more growth you will experience, and as you mature, the more you will cultivate others around you.

It's vital to understand that the thoughts, feelings, and actions you express in life are what you are projecting out into the atmosphere. So, what you think and do today shapes your tomorrow.

POWER IN SERVICE

In life, I have learned that you get back what you put in. Therefore, the forces, people, and circumstances you attract are a reflection of what you have given.

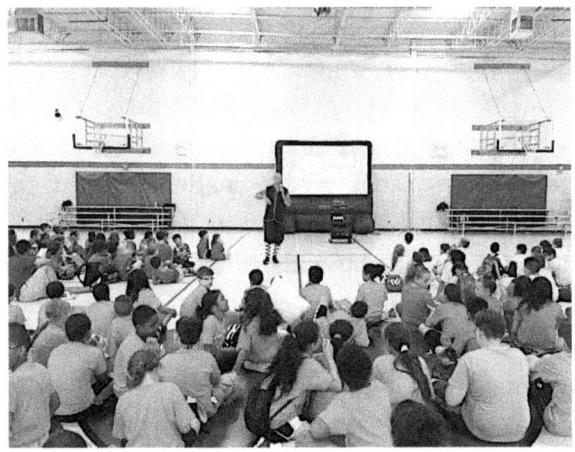

You will never have power if you violate nature's laws. And you may face dire consequences of bad karma if you violate them. For example, if you manipulate people into serving you for your benefit, you will find that any manipulative power obtained is passive and temporary because you do not gain spiritual strength. As a result, your power and privileges will not last. Going against nature will force you back, because what you give is what you are given.

The attainment of power is nature's reward for obeying her laws. If you attempt to attain power without earning it, you will violate these laws. We were put on earth to serve each other. *What good is having power if you don't do anything with it that benefits others?*

If you obtain power and only use it for your benefit, nature will step in and take it away. Thinking of ways to serve others enables you to grow physically, intellectually, and spiritually, and obtain more influence, abundance, and power.

We must serve each other. When nature recognizes your service, she gifts you with more power. **We get what we give.** The more service we provide, the more power we accumulate. If you earn something without learning how to manage it and distribute it to others beneficially, then it will be taken away. Everything has its price, and you will pay that price no matter what. That is natural law.

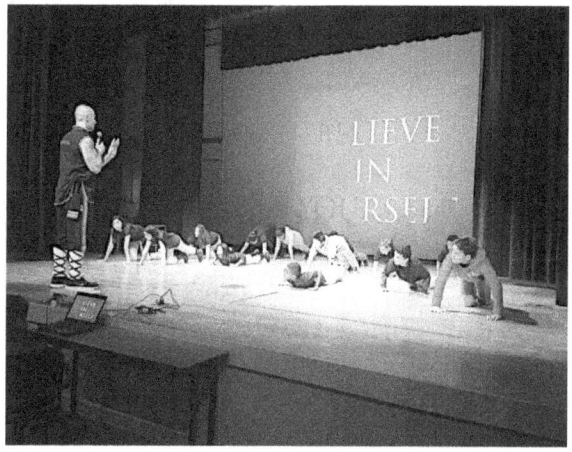

Those who think life is unfair and always want something without giving in return are rendered powerless and always will be.

Almost everything comes into our life from what we have within ourselves. This force projects our energy through the atmosphere and resonates with the natural laws, and this is what brings us the forces, people, and experiences that harmonize with our own thoughts and actions.

There is no guesswork here, no such thing as miracles or luck. You are either attracting or repelling energy. Positive energy is omnipotent and negative energy is impotent. It is your consciousness that determines your results in life. All of these circumstances can provide you with the power you need if you know how to manage them.

There are millions of ways that life can distract us, and you may think you don't have sufficient time and effort to better your present situation. However, if you keep studying and practicing, you will find that your life starts to get better in all areas.

In closing, I wish to express that those who seek power must learn that they will never obtain it unless they serve others first. **Power is found in service.** The more you give, the more you get back. This natural law is a recurring theme in life, not just in this book.

For a martial artist, a higher state of awareness is having the wisdom to transfer faith and positive energy into others. This means that you hurt yourself by hurting others. You hurt others by not being of service to them. **Remember, the critical part of wellbeing is well-doing.** A true warrior helps others first at all costs. This golden rule is the undeniable Shaolin way.

GATE 3 KEY POINTS

1. Life starts with breathing, which is the key to power.
2. Power is essential for all possession, all achievement, and all success.
3. There are three planes of power: physical, mental, and spiritual.
4. We obtain power in the physical plane through exercise and practice.
5. We receive power in the mental plane through meditation and a harmonious alliance with others.
6. We gain power in the spiritual plane from connecting to the source of all energy in the world within.
7. In the physical plane, the body is at its best through exercise and when thermal energy is flowing freely and naturally.
8. In the mental plane, power generates through daily meditation.
9. In the spiritual plane, providing service increases your power.
10. Because of an inflexible natural law, what you give is what you get.

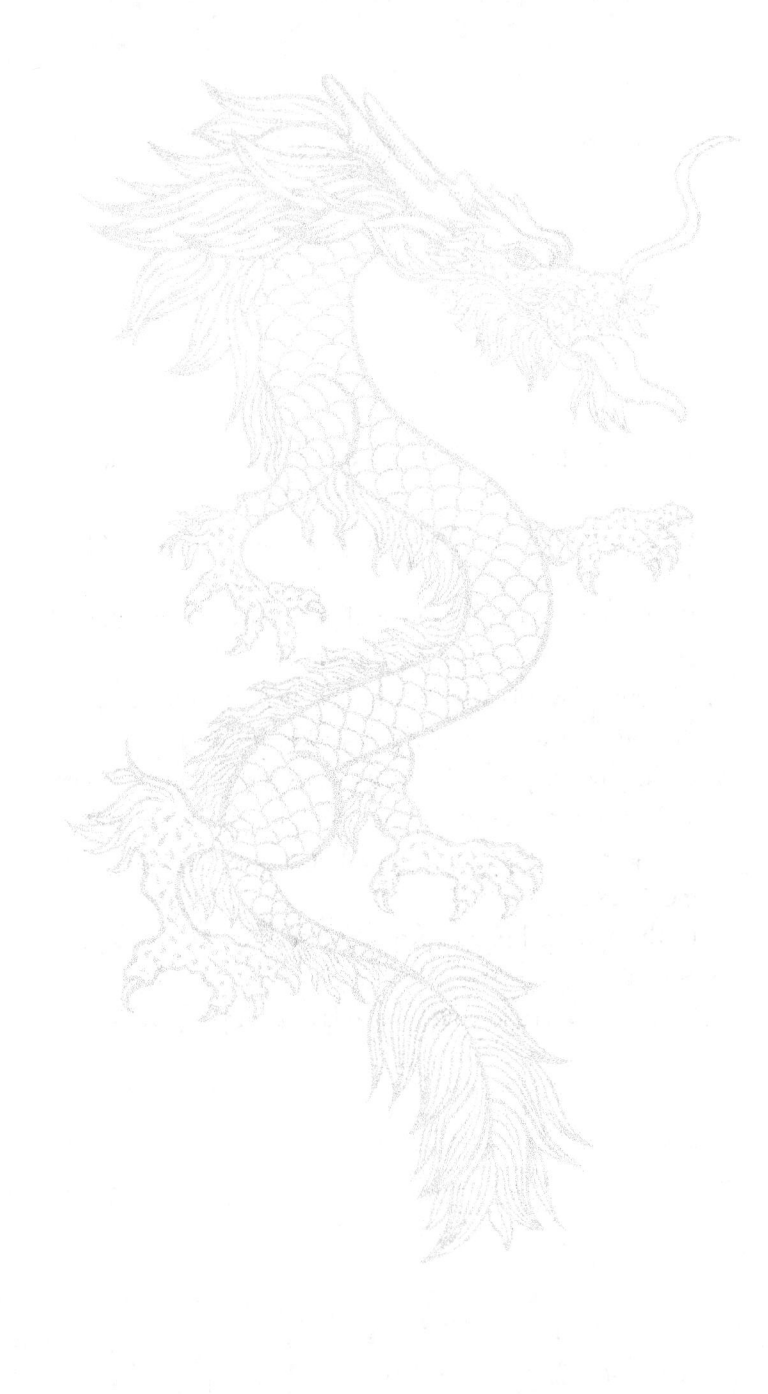

EPILOGUE

You have just finished reading the first book in a series of three. After you have thoroughly digested the material within this manifesto, you will ultimately have learned that the body only represents a part of your total power. This part is objective, dealing with the physical, outside world.

To increase your overall strength in all areas of your life, study the other two factors thoroughly: the mind and spirit. These will be detailed in the next two volumes in this series.

This book's primary focus was on the body and enhancing its connection to the physical side of life. Book two will focus on the mind and introduce the attributes that will enhance your overall mental wellbeing. The purpose of book two is to induce the state of mind that will complement the physical attributes attained after reading this book to acquire the ultimate mind-body connection.

For more information on Denis Ark and any upcoming news or events, please visit www.invincibleark.com.

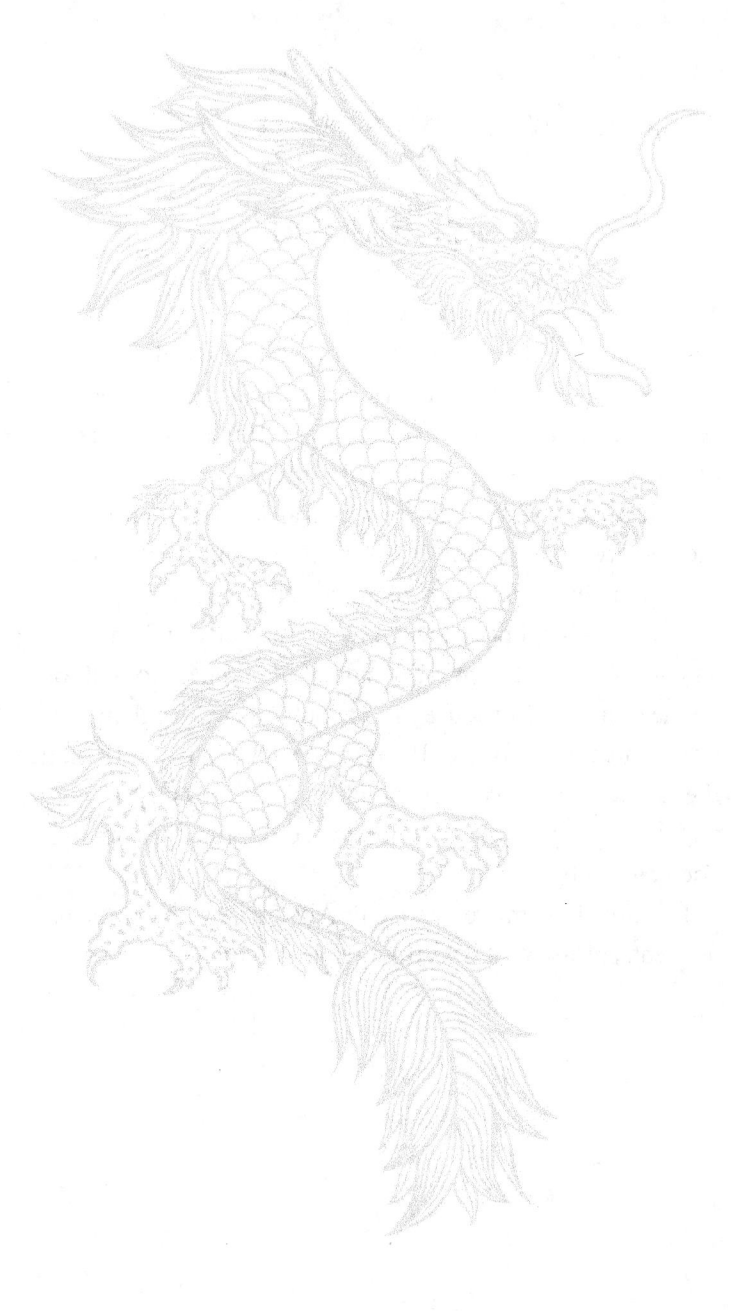

ABOUT THE AUTHOR

Denis Ark is a *Masters of the Martial Arts:* Hall of Fame Martial Artist (Atlantic City, N.J. 2019), Certified Fitness Trainer (CFT), and Certified Strength & Conditioning Specialist (CSCS). He is the owner/head instructor of *Invincible Ark Fitness & Martial Arts.* He has dedicated his life to the study and promotion of martial arts, fitness, and health and wellness, serving others by helping them change their lives for the better in every aspect.

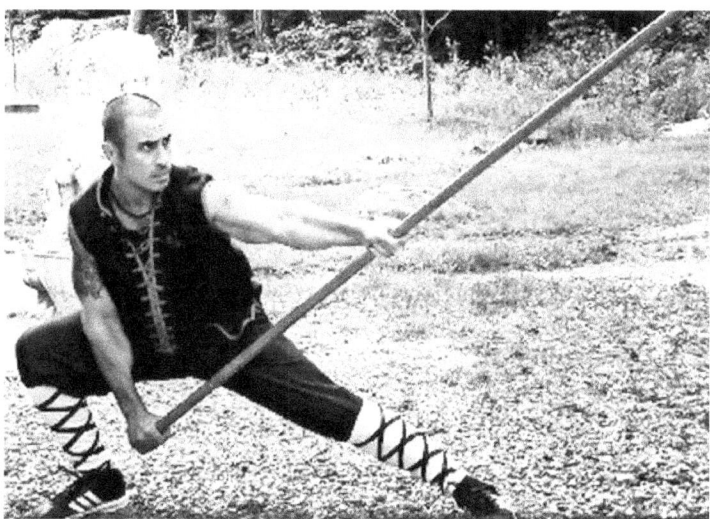

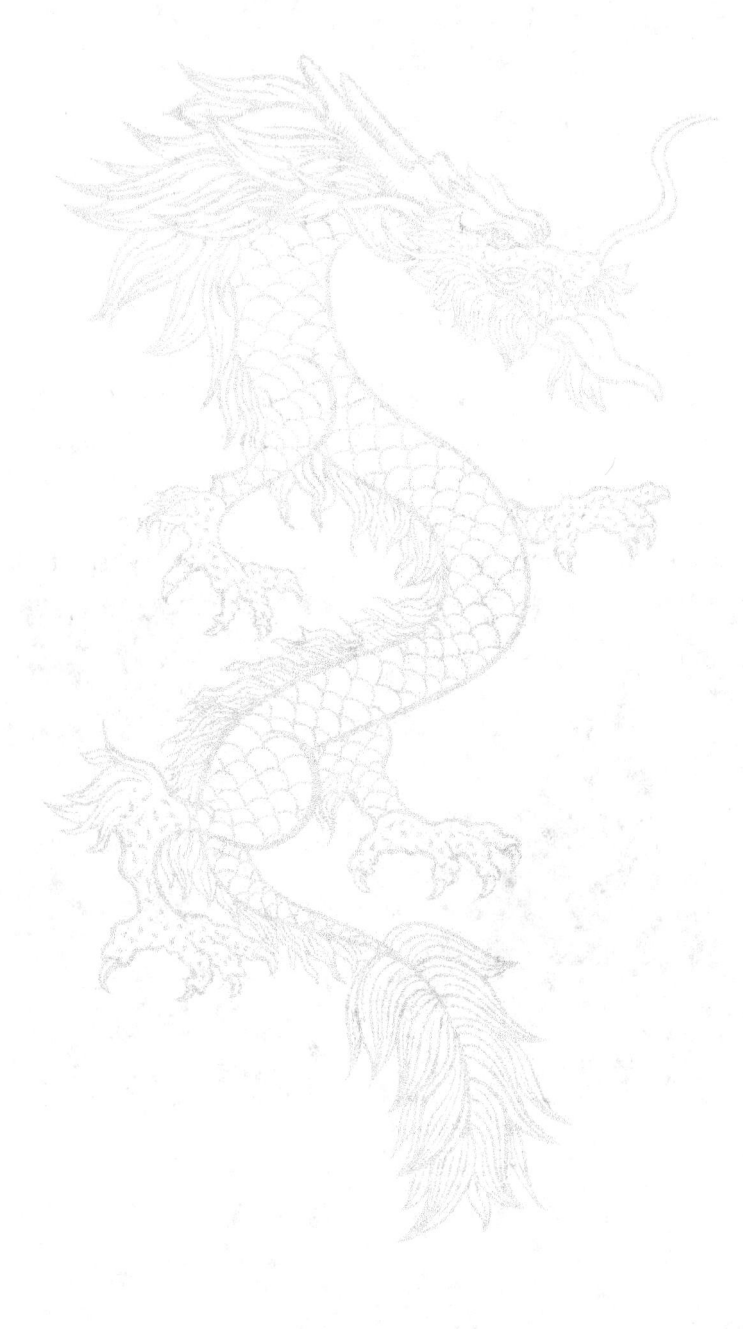

ENDNOTES

PREFACE

1. Daisetz Teitaro Suzuki, *Manual Of Zen Buddhism* (New York, USA: Grove Press Inc. 1960).

2. Charles W. Kenn, *A Brief History of Gung Fu* (Copyright 1963 by Charles W. Kenn. Honolulu, Hawaii, 1963).

3. Miyamoto Musashi, *The Book Of Five Rings: Gorin No Sho*. Translation and Commentary by Nikon Services Corporation: Bradford J. Brown, Yuko Kashiwagi, William H. Barrett, and Eisuke Sasagawa. (New York, Toronto, London, Sydney, Auckland: Bantam Books. 1982).

4. Miyamoto Musashi, Stephen F. Kaufman, *The Book Of Five Rings: The definitive interpretation of Miyamoto Musashi's classic book of strategy*. (Tokyo, Rutland, Vermont, Singapore: Tuttle Publishing, 1994).

5. Miyamoto Musashi, *The Book Of Five Rings* (Bantam Books.) TIME Magazine – Critic Review. 1982.

6. Newsweek Magazine. *Bruce Lee: 75 Years of the Dragon,* (New York City, New York USA: Dev Pragad. 2015).

7. Bruce, Lee, M. Uyehara, *Bruce Lee's Fighting Method: Skill in Techniques Vol. 3*. (Santa Clarita, California USA: O'Hara Publications, Inc. Copyright 1977, by Linda Lee. 1973).

8. Wei Lo, Hsiang Wu Chia, Raymond Chow, *The Big Boss*. Film. Golden Harvest Productions. Hong Kong. 1971.

9. Wei Lo, Raymond Chow, *Fist of Fury*. Film. Golden Harvest Productions. Hong Kong. 1972.

10. Bruce Lee, Raymond Chow, *Way of the Dragon*. Film. Concord Production Inc. Hong Kong. 1972.

11. Robert Clouse, Michael Allin, Bruce Lee, *Enter the Dragon*. Film. Warner Bros. 1972.

12   Alex Proyas, James O'Barr, David J. Schow, John Shirley, *The Crow*. Film. Miramax. 1994.

13   Newsweek Magazine, *Bruce Lee: 75 Years of the Dragon*, (New York City, New York USA: Dev Pragad. 2015).

INTRODUCTION

14   Britannica, "Sir Edmund Hillary," Britannica.com, September 11, 2021, Accessed September 11, 2021, https://www.britannica.com/biography/Edmund-Hillary

GATE 1: MARTIAL ARTS

15   Napoleon Hill, *Outwitting The Devil: The Secret to Freedom and Success* (New York, USA: Sterling Publishing Co., Inc. 2011).

16   Earl Nightingale *Think and Grow Rich – Audiobook*, Narrated by Earl Nightingale (USA. Brilliance Audio. 1937).

17   Thomas Carlyle, The Beasts of Ephesus. (1892).

CHAPTER 1: WHAT ARE MARTIAL ARTS?

18   Napoleon Hill, *Think and Grow Rich* (Produced by Books-A-Million: Sweet Water Press 2012, original 1938).

CHAPTER 2: VISION QUEST

19   Sun Tzu, Stephen F. Kaufman, *The Art Of War: The definitive interpretation of Sun Tzu's classic book of strategy for the martial artist*. (Tokyo, Rutland, Vermont, Boston: Tuttle Publishing. 1996).

20   Miyamoto Musashi, Stephen F. Kaufman, *The Book Of Five Rings: The definitive interpretation of Miyamoto Musashi's classic book of strategy*. (Tokyo, Rutland, Vermont, Singapore: Tuttle Publishing, 1994).

21   Ralph Waldo Emerson, Essays and Poems by Ralph Waldo Emerson: With an Introduction and Notes by Peter Norberg. (New York, New York USA: Barnes & Noble Books. 2004).

22   Charles F. Haanel, The Master Key System. (Printed in the USA: No Publishing Company listed 1912).

23   Wallace, D. Wattles, How To What You Want. (USA: Originally Published in 1907. JonRose Publishing, 2016).

24   Napoleon Hill, How To Raise Your Own Salary. (Chicago, Illinois USA: Napoleon Hill Associates – A Division of W. Clement Stone Enterprises. 1953).

25   Jwing-Ming Yang, The Root Of Chinese Qigong: Secrets Of Health, Longevity, and Enlightenment (YMAA Publication Center, 1997).

26 Charles W. Kenn, A Brief History of Gung Fu (Copyright 1963 by Charles W. Kenn. Honolulu, Hawaii, 1963).

27 Bruce Lee Quotes, BrainyQuote.com, BrainyMedia Inc, 2021, Accessed September 11, 2021, www.brainyquote.com/citation/quotes/bruce_lee_413509

CHAPTER 5: THE WARRIOR SPIRIT

28 Sifu Bill Fong, "History of Hung Ga and Shaolin," FongsHungGa.com, Accessed September 11, 2021, https://www.fongshungga.com/about

29 Ping Ngai, Chen Long, Rongjin, Kung Fu Quest: Shaolin. Documentary. 2016.

30 Daisetz Teitaro Suzuki, Manual Of Zen Buddhism (New York, USA: Grove Press Inc. 1960).

GATE 2: THE FOUR FACTORS OF FITNESS

31 Miyamoto Musashi, *The Book Of Five Rings: Gorin No Sho*. Translation and Commentary by Nikon Services Corporation: Bradford J. Brown, Yuko Kashiwagi, William H. Barrett, and Eisuke Sasagawa. (New York, Toronto, London, Sydney, Auckland: Bantam Books. 1982).

32 Henry Gray, F.R.S. (1901, 1995). *Gray's Anatomy*: 15th Edition. (New York, New York USA: Barnes & Noble Books).

33 Tim Newman, Han Seunggu, M.D. (2017). *All About the Central Nervous Systems*. MedicalNewsToday.com

34 Henry Gray, F.R.S. (1901, 1995). *Gray's Anatomy*: 15th Edition. (New York, New York USA: Barnes & Noble Books).

CHAPTER 6: STRENGTH

35 MK Yau, "Tai Chi exercise and the improvement of health and well-being in older adults," PubMed.Gov National Institutes Of Health, 2008, Accessed September 11, 2021, https://pubmed.ncbi.nlm.nih.gov/18487895/

36 Jin Jing Zhong, *Authentic Shaolin Heritage: Training Methods of 72 Arts of Shaolin*. Translation Editor Andrew Timofeevich. Translated by Wang Ke Ze, Leonid Serbin, Ekatarina Buga, & Oleg Korshunov. (USA. CreateSpace, Copyright 2004, by Andrew Timofeevich, original 1934).

CHAPTER 7: FLEXIBILITY

37 Frederick C. Hatfield MSS, PhD. *Fitness: The Complete Guide*. (Carpinteria, California: International Sports Sciences Association 2013).

38 Bruce. Lee, M. Uyehara, *Bruce Lee's Fighting Method: Skill in Techniques Vol. 3*. Copyright 1977, by Linda Lee, (Santa Clarita, California USA: O'Hara Publications, Inc. 1973).

39   James Y. Lee, (1957, 1958, 1962, 1963). *Modern Kung-Fu Karate: Iron, Poison Hand Training Book 1.* (USA. No Publisher listed. Third revised Edition 1963).

CHAPTER 8: CONDITIONING

40   Thomas D. Fahey EdD, *Strength and Conditioning* (Carpinteria, California: International Sports Sciences Association. 2013).

41   Frederick C. Hatfield MSS, PhD. *Fitness: The Complete Guide* (Carpinteria, California: International Sports Sciences Association. 2013).

42   Arnold Schwarzenegger, Bill Dobbins, *The New Encyclopedia of Modern Bodybuilding* (New York City, New York USA: Simon & Schuster. 1995, 1998).

43   Frederick C. Hatfield MSS, PhD. *Fitness: The Complete Guide.* (Carpinteria, California: International Sports Sciences Association 2013).

44   Frederick C. Hatfield MSS, PhD. *Fitness: The Complete Guide.* (Carpinteria, California: International Sports Sciences Association 2013).

45   Thomas D. Fahey EdD. *Strength and Conditioning.* (Carpinteria, California: International Sports Sciences Association 2013).

46   Frederick C. Hatfield MSS, PhD. *Fitness: The Complete Guide.* (Carpinteria, California: International Sports Sciences Association 2013).

CHAPTER 9: NUTRITION

47   Ralph Waldo Emerson, *Essays and Poems by Ralph Waldo Emerson: With an Introduction and Notes by Peter Norberg* (New York, New York USA: Barnes & Noble Books 2004).

48   Frederick C. Hatfield MSS, PhD. *Fitness: The Complete Guide* (Carpinteria, California: International Sports Sciences Association 2013).

49   Natural Food Pantry, "No Disease Can Exist In An Alkaline Environment," June 16, 2017. Accessed September 11, 2021. https://naturalfoodpantry.ca/blogs/mind-body/no-disease-can-exist-in-an-alkaline-environment

50   Otto Heinrich Warburg MD, "Otto Heinrich Warburg," Wikepedia.com, Accessed September 11, 2021, https://en.wikipedia.org/wiki/Otto_Heinrich_Warburg

51   Ping Ngai, Chen Long, Rongjin, *Kung Fu Quest: Shaolin.* Documentary. 2016.

52   Britannica, "Chakra," Britannica.com, Accessed September 11, 2021, https://www.britannica.com/topic/chakra

53   Wikipedia, "Traditional Chinese Medicine," Wikipedia.com, Accessed September 11, 2021, https://en.wikipedia.org/wiki/Traditional_Chinese_medicine

54   Wikipedia, "Acupuncture," Wikipedia.com, Accessed September 11, 2021, https://en.wikipedia.org/wiki/Acupuncture

55 Academy of Nutrition and Dietetics, "Vegetarian and Special Diets," EatRight. org, Accessed September 11, 2021, https://www.eatright.org/food/nutrition/vegetarian-and-special-diets

56 Theresa Fung ScD, RD, LDN, Sharon Palmer RDN, *Healthy Eating: A guide to the new nutrition* (Harvard Medical School. Harvard Health Publishing 2016).

57 Frederick C. Hatfield, MSS, PhD. (2013). *Fitness: The Complete Guide*. (Carpinteria, California: International Sports Sciences Association).

58 Sandra Cabot, MD, "Liver Doctor," LiverDoctor.org, Accessed September 11, 2021, https://www.liverdoctor.com/about-dr-sandra-cabot/

59 Susan Bernstein, Minesh Khatri MD, "What is Toxic Liver Disease or Hepatotoxicity," WebMD.com, May 29, 2020, Accessed September 11, 2021, https://www.webmd.com/hepatitis/toxic-liver-disease

60 NCBI, "LiverTox: Clinical and Research Information on Drug Induced Liver Injury," " NonSteroidal Anti-inflammatory Drugs NSAID's," NCBI.gov, March 18, 2020, Accessed September 11,2021, https://www.ncbi.nlm.nih.gov/books/NBK548614/

61 NLM, "Nonsteroidal anti-inflammatory drug – induced liver injury – control study in primary care," PubMed.gov, April 18, 2004, Accessed September 11, 2021, https://pubmed.ncbi.nlm.nih.gov/15066135/

62 University of South Alabama, "Drugs and Health Risks," SouthAlabama.edu, Accessed September 11, 2021, https://www.southalabama.edu/departments/counseling/healthrisks.html

63 FDA, "Acetaminophen Information," FDA.gov, November 14, 2017, Accessed September 11, 2021, https://www.fda.gov/drugs/information-drug-class/acetaminophen-information

64 Sandra Cabot, MD, "Why Your Liver Needs a Cleanse," LiverDoctor. org, Accessed September 11, 2021, https://www.liverdoctor.com/part-1-compelling-reasons-why-your-liver-needs-a-cleanse/

65 Helen West, RD, "7 Science-Based of Milk Thistle," Healthline.com, January 19, 2018, Accessed September 11, 2021, https://www.healthline.com/nutrition/milk-thistle-benefits

66 Maria Valentina Ignat, "Medicinal Value of Chicory," Encyclopedia.pub, Accessed September 11, 2021, https://encyclopedia.pub/9424

67 Healthline, "5 Emerging Benefits and Uses of Yarrow Tea," EcoWatch.com, December 22, 2019, Accessed September 11, 2021, https://www.ecowatch.com/yarrow-tea-health-benefits-2641669777.html#toggle-gdpr

68 SD Desai, BS Patil, PS Kanthe, "Effect of ethanolic extract of terminalia arjuna on liver functions and histopathology of liver in albino rats fed with hyperlipidemic

diet," 1MG.com, August 24, 2015, Accessed September 11, 2021, https://www.1mg.com/ayurveda/arjuna-102

69   PubMed, "The Role of Tamarix gallica Leaves Extract in Liver Injury Induced by Rifampicin Plus Isoniazid in Sprague Dawley Rats," PubMed.gov, January 2, 2018, Accessed September 11, 2021, https://pubmed.ncbi.nlm.nih.gov/28459346/

70   Ansley Hill, RD, "13 Potential Health Benefits of Dandelion," Healthline.com, July 18, 2018, Accessed September 11, 2021, https://www.healthline.com/nutrition/dandelion-benefits#TOC_TITLE_HDR_5

71   NCBI, NIH, "Anticancer Properties of Graviola (*Annona muricata*): A Comprehensive Mechanistic Review," US National Library of Medicine, National Institute of Health, NCBI.NLM.NIH.gov, July 30, 2018, Accessed September 11, 2021, https://www.ncbi.nlm.nih.gov/pmc/articles/PMC6091294/

72   Kevin Trudeau, *Natural Cures: They Don't Want You To Know About*. (Alliance Pub Group Inc., 2005).

73   Richard Smith, "Let Food Be Thy Medicine…" US National Library of Medicine, National Institute of Health, NCBI.NLM.NIH.gov, January 24, 2004, Accessed September 11, 2021, https://www.ncbi.nlm.nih.gov/pmc/articles/PMC318470/

74   Richard Shulze ND, MH. *Dr. Shulze's 20 Powerful Steps to a Healthier Life* (California USA: Natural Healing Publications 2010).

75   Nicholas Wade, "Your Body Is Younger Than You Think," New York Times, nytimes.com, August 2, 2005, Accessed September 11, 2021, https://www.nytimes.com/2005/08/02/science/your-body-is-younger-than-you-think.html

76   Douglas Heaven, "Nuclear Bomb Tests Reveal Brain Regeneration In Humans," NewScientist.com, June 7, 2013, Accessed September 11, 2021, https://www.newscientist.com/article/dn23665-nuclear-bomb-tests-reveal-brain-regeneration-in-humans/

77   National Institute of Diabetes and Digestive and Kidney Diseases, "Health Risks of Overweight & Obesity," NIDDK.NIH.gov, February 2018, Accessed September 11, 2021, https://www.niddk.nih.gov/health-information/weight-management/adult-overweight-obesity/health-risks

78   Kelly Bramlet Blackburn, "What Happens When You Overeat," The University of Texas MD Anderson Cancer Center, MDanderson.org, February 2018, Accessed September 11, 2021, https://www.mdanderson.org/publications/focused-on-health/What-happens-when-you-overeat.h23Z1592202.html

79   PubMed, "Associations among binge eating behavior patterns and gastrointestinal symptoms: a population-based study," US National Library of Medicine, National Institute of Health, NCBI.NLM.NIH.gov, January 3, 2009, Accessed September 11, 2021, https://www.ncbi.nlm.nih.gov/pmc/articles/PMC2754813/

80   National Institute of Health, "Risk in Red Meat?" NIH.gov, March 26, 2012, Accessed September 11, 2021, https://www.nih.gov/news-events/nih-research-matters/risk-red-meat

81   National Institute of Health, "Parasites associated with pork and pork products," PubMed.gov, August 16, 1997. Accessed September 11,2021, https://pubmed.ncbi.nlm.nih.gov/9501363/

82   USDA, "Food and Nutrition, Dietary Health" US Department of Agriculture, USDA.gov, Accessed September 11, 2021, https://www.usda.gov/topics/food-and-nutrition/dietary-health

83   CDC, "Parasites – Trichinellosis Epidemiology & Risk Factors," Center for Disease Control & Prevention, CDC.gov, November 15, 2019, Accessed September 11, 2021, https://www.cdc.gov/parasites/trichinellosis/epi.html

84   PubMed, "Potential Animal Health Hazards of Pork and Pork Products," National Institute of Health, PubMed.NCBI.NLM.NIH.gov, April 16, 1997, Accessed September 11, 2021, https://pubmed.ncbi.nlm.nih.gov/9329109/

85   Josh Axe, MD, *"Why You Should Avoid Pork,"* Evidence Based Nutrition: DrAxe.com, October 31, 2016, Accessed September 11, 2021, https://draxe.com/nutrition/why-you-should-avoid-pork/

86   Kevin Trudeau, *Your Wish Is Your Command.* Audio CD. (Publisher: The Global Information Network 2009).

87   PMC Labs, "Poultry and Livestock Exposure and Cancer Risk among Farmers in the Agricultural Health Study," National Institute of Health, PubMed.NCBI.NLM.NIH.gov, March 10, 2012, Accessed September 11, 2021, https://www.ncbi.nlm.nih.gov/pmc/articles/PMC3337970/

88   Ping Ngai, Chen Long, Rongjin, *Kung Fu Quest: Shaolin.* Documentary. 2016.

89   Heidi Godman, "Think Fast When Kids Want Fast Food," January 31, 2013, Harvard Health, Health.Harvard.edu. Accessed September 11, 2021, https://www.health.harvard.edu/blog/think-fast-when-kids-want-fast-food-201301315846

90   WCRF "Limit Fast Foods" World Cancer Research Fund, WCRF.org, 2018, Accessed September 11, 2021, https://www.wcrf.org/dietandcancer/limit-fast-foods/

91   WCRF "Limit Red and Processed Meats" World Cancer Research Fund, WCRF.org, 2018, Accessed September 11, 2021, https://www.wcrf.org/dietandcancer/limit-red-and-processed-meat/

92   WCRF "Cancer Prevention Recommendations" World Cancer Research Fund, WCRF.org, 2018, Accessed September 11, 2021, https://www.wcrf.org/diet-and-cancer/cancer-prevention-recommendations

93   Frederick C. Hatfield MSS, PhD. *Fitness: The Complete Guide.* (Carpinteria, California: International Sports Sciences Association 2013).

94   PubMed, "The Sweet Dangers of Added Sugars," National Institute of Health, PubMed.NCBI.NLM.NIH.gov, June 20, 2019, Accessed September 11, 2021, https://pubmed.ncbi.nlm.nih.gov/31246081/

GATE 3: INTERNAL ENERGY

95   Wikipedia, "Meridian (Traditional Chinese Medicine)" Wikipedia.com, Accessed September 11, 2021, https://en.wikipedia.org/wiki/Meridian_(Chinese_medicine)

96   Ralph Waldo Emerson, *Essays and Poems by Ralph Waldo Emerson: With an Introduction and Notes by Peter Norberg* (New York, New York USA: Barnes & Noble Books 2004).

97   Charles F. Haanel, *The Master Key System*. (Printed in the USA: No Publishing Company listed 1912).

98   Manly Palmer Hall, *Animals and the Cosmic Order: Lectures On Ancient Philosophy by Manly P. Hall*. (Audio Lecture, 1929).

99   Charles F. Haanel, *The Master Key System* (Printed in the USA: No Publishing Company listed 1912).

CHAPTER 10: POWER IN PROVIDENCE

100 Three Initiates, *The Kybalion* (Tarcher Perigree, Imprint of Penguin House LLC, 2018, original 1908).

101 Charles F. Haanel, *The Master Key System* (Printed in the USA: No Publishing Company listed 1912).

102 Bruce H. Lipton Ph.D., *The Biology Of Belief: Unleashing the Power of Consciousness, Matter, & Miracles* (Carlsbad, California, New York City, London, Sydney, Johannesburg, Vancouver, Hong Kong, and New Delhi: Hay House, Inc. 2005).

CHAPTER 12: POWER IN PRACTICE

103 Miyamoto Musashi, Stephen F. Kaufman, *The Book Of Five Rings: The definitive interpretation of Miyamoto Musashi's classic book of strategy* (Tokyo, Rutland, Vermont, Singapore: Tuttle Publishing, 1994).

104 Daisetz Teitaro Suzuki, *Manual Of Zen Buddhism* (New York, USA: Grove Press Inc. 1960).

CHAPTER 13: PHYSICAL POWER

105 Julia Seton M.D., *Psychology Of The Solar Plexus And The Subconscious Mind* (New York: Edward J. Clode, 1914).

106 Julia Seton, M.D., *Psychology Of The Solar Plexus And The Subconscious Mind* (New York: Edward J. Clode, 1914).

107 Charles F. Haanel, *The Master Key System*. (Printed in the USA: No Publishing Company listed, 1912).

108 Julia Seton MD, *Psychology Of The Solar Plexus And The Subconscious Mind* (New York: Edward J. Clode. 1914).

CHAPTER 14: MENTAL POWER

109 Sai Wing Lam, *Iron Thread*. Authorized Translation by Jyu Yu Jaai. Hong Kong 1957. Copyright Compiled and edited by Andrew Timofeevich. Translated by Wang Ke Ze, Leonid Serbin, & Oleg Korshunov. (USA. CreateSpace 2002, by Andrew Timofeevich, original 1932).

110 Yang, Jwing-Ming. *The Root Of Chinese Qigong: Secrets Of Health, Longevity, and Enlightenment*. YMAA Publication Center. 1997.

111 Trudeau, Kevin. *Your Wish Is Your Command*. Audio CD. Publisher: The Global Information Network. 2009.

CHAPTER 15: SPIRITUAL POWER

112 Pierre Teilhard De Chardin, Quote Investigator, Accessed September 11, 2021, https://quoteinvestigator.com/tag/pierre-teilhard-de-chardin/

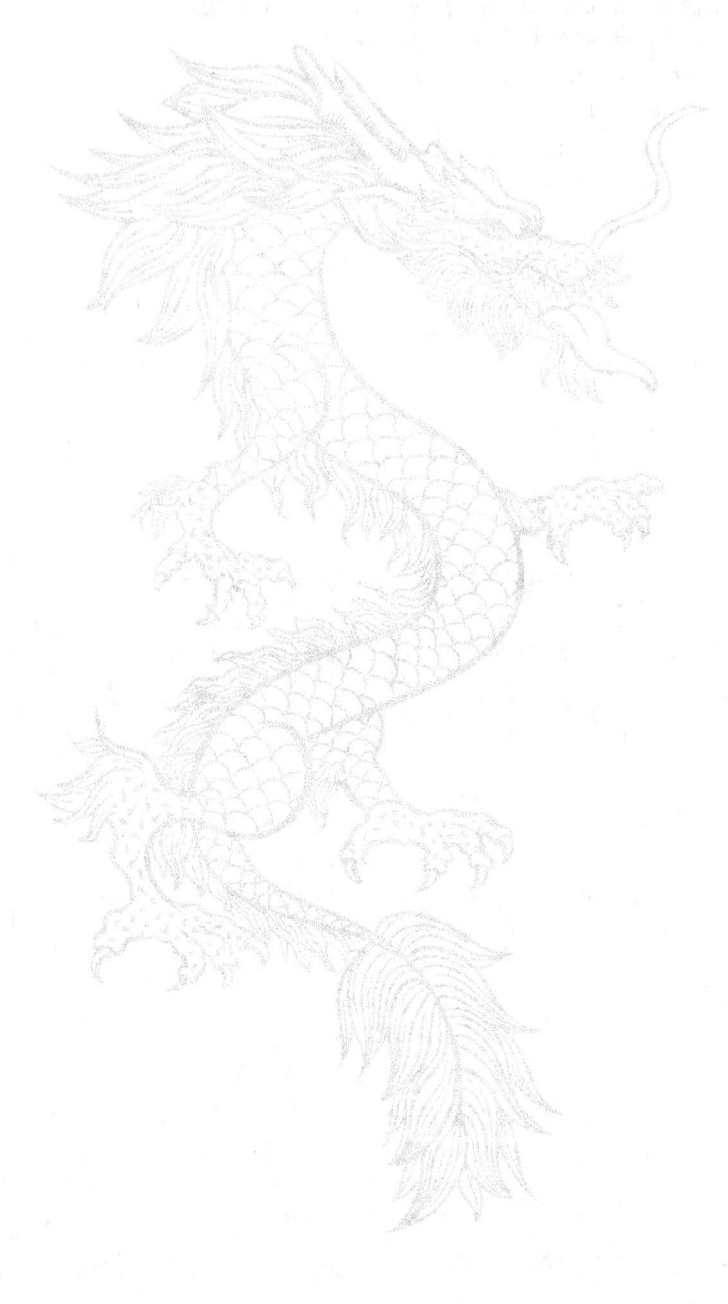

REFERENCES

Academy of Nutrition and Dietetics. "Vegetarian and Special Diets." EatRight.org. Accessed September 11, 2021. https://www.eatright.org/food/nutrition/vegetarian-and-special-diets

Axe, Josh, M.D. "*Why You Should Avoid Pork.*" Evidence Based Nutrition: DrAxe.com. October 31, 2016. Accessed September 11, 2021. https://draxe.com/nutrition/why-you-should-avoid-pork/

Bernstein, Susan. Khatri, Minesh MD. "What is Toxic Liver Disease or Hepatotoxicity." WebMD.com. May 29, 2020. Accessed September 11, 2021. https://www.webmd.com/hepatitis/toxic-liver-disease

Blackburn, Kelly Bramlet. "What Happens When You Overeat." The University of Texas MD Anderson Cancer Center. MDanderson.org. February 2018. Accessed September 11, 2021. https://www.mdanderson.org/publications/focused-on-health/What-happens-when-you-overeat.h23Z1592202.html

Britannica. "Chakra." Britannica.com. Accessed September 11, 2021. https://www.britannica.com/topic/chakra

Britannica. "Sir Edmund Hillary." Britannica.com. September 11, 2021. Accessed September 11, 2021. https://www.britannica.com/biography/Edmund-Hillary

Bruce Lee Quotes. BrainyQuote.com. BrainyMedia Inc. 2021. Accessed September 11, 2021. www.brainyquote.com/citation/quotes/bruce_lee_413509

Cabot, Sandra MD. "Why Your Liver Needs a Cleanse." LiverDoctor.org. Accessed September 11, 2021. https://www.liverdoctor.com/part-1-compelling-reasons-why-your-liver-needs-a-cleanse/

CDC. "Parasites – Trichinellosis Epidemiology & Risk Factors." Center for Disease Control & Prevention. CDC.gov. November 15, 2019. Accessed September 11, 2021. https://www.cdc.gov/parasites/trichinellosis/epi.html

De Chardin, Pierre Teilhard. Quote Investigator. Accessed September 11, 2021. https://quoteinvestigator.com/tag/pierre-teilhard-de-chardin/

Desai, SD. Patil, BS. Kanthe, PS. "Effect of ethanolic extract of terminalia arjuna on liver functions and histopathology of liver in albino rats fed with hyperlipidemic diet." 1MG.com. August 24, 2015. Accessed September 11, 2021. https://www.1mg.com/ayurveda/arjuna-102

Emerson, Ralph Waldo. *Essays and Poems by Ralph Waldo Emerson: With an Introduction and Notes by Peter Norberg.* New York, New York USA: Barnes & Noble Books. 2004.

Fahey, Thomas D., EdD. *Strength and Conditioning.* Carpinteria, California: International Sports Sciences Association. 2013.

FDA. "Acetaminophen Information." FDA.gov. November 14, 2017. Accessed September 11, 2021. https://www.fda.gov/drugs/information-drug-class/acetaminophen-information

Fong, Sifu Bill. "History of Hung Ga and Shaolin." FongsHungGa.com. Accessed September 11, 2021. https://www.fongshungga.com/about

Fung, Theresa ScD, RD, LDN. Palmer, Sharon, RDN. *Healthy Eating: A guide to the new nutrition.* Harvard Medical School. Harvard Health Publishing. 2016.

Godman, Heidi. "Think Fast When Kids Want Fast Food." January 31, 2013. Harvard Health. Health.Harvard.edu. Accessed September 11, 2021. https://www.health.harvard.edu/blog/think-fast-when-kids-want-fast-food-201301315846

Gray, Henry, F.R.S. *Gray's Anatomy*: 15th Edition. New York, New York USA: Barnes & Noble Books. 1901, 1995.

Haanel, Charles F. *The Master Key System.* Printed in the USA: No Publishing Company listed. 1912.

Hatfield, Frederick C., MSS, PhD. *Fitness: The Complete Guide.* Carpinteria, California: International Sports Sciences Association. 2013.

Healthline. "5 Emerging Benefits and Uses of Yarrow Tea." EcoWatch.com. December 22, 2019. Accessed September 11, 2021. https://www.ecowatch.com/yarrow-tea-health-benefits-2641669777.html#toggle-gdpr

Heaven, Douglas. "Nuclear Bomb Tests Reveal Brain Regeneration In Humans." NewScientist.com. June 7, 2013. Accessed September 11, 2021. https://www.newscientist.com/article/dn23665-nuclear-bomb-tests-reveal-brain-regeneration-in-humans/

Hill, Ansley RD. "13 Potential Health Benefits of Dandelion." Healthline.com. July 18, 2018. Accessed September 11, 2021. https://www.healthline.com/nutrition/dandelion-benefits#TOC_TITLE_HDR_5

Hill, Napoleon. *How To Raise Your Own Salary.* Chicago, Illinois USA: Napoleon Hill Associates – A Division of W. Clement Stone Enterprises. 1953.

Hill, Napoleon. *Outwitting The Devil: The Secret to Freedom and Success.* New York, USA: Sterling Publishing Co., Inc. 2011.

Hill, Napoleon. *Think and Grow Rich.* Produced by Books-A-Million: Sweet Water Press 1938, 2012.

Ignat, Maria Valentina. "Medicinal Value of Chicory." Encyclopedia.pub. Accessed September 11, 2021. https://encyclopedia.pub/9424

Jin, Jing Zhong. *Authentic Shaolin Heritage: Training Methods of 72 Arts of Shaolin.* Translation Editor Andrew Timofeevich. Translated by Wang Ke Ze, Leonid Serbin, Ekatarina Buga, & Oleg Korshunov. USA. CreateSpace. Copyright 2004 by Andrew Timofeevich. 1934.

Kenn, Charles W. A Brief History of Gung Fu. Copyright 1963 by Charles W. Kenn. Honolulu, Hawaii. 1963.

Kong, Bucksam. *The Tiger/Crane Form of Hung Gar Kung Fu.* Twentieth Printing 2008. Copyright 1983. O'Hara Publications, Inc. 1983.

Lam, Sai Wing. *Iron Thread.* Authorized Translation by Jyu Yu Jaai. Hong Kong 1957. Copyright (2002) by Andrew Timofeevich. Compiled and edited by Andrew Timofeevich. Translated by Wang Ke Ze, Leonid Serbin, & Oleg Korshunov. USA. CreateSpace. *1932.*

Lee, Bruce. Uyehara, M. *Bruce Lee's Fighting Method: Basic Training Vol. 2.* Copyright (1977) by Linda Lee. Santa Clarita, California USA: O'Hara Publications, Inc. 1973.

Lee, Bruce., Uyehara, M. *Bruce Lee's Fighting Method: Skill in Techniques Vol. 3.* Copyright (1977) by Linda Lee. Santa Clarita, California USA: O'Hara Publications, Inc. 1973.

Lee, James Y. (1957, 1958, 1962, 1963). *Modern Kung-Fu Karate: Iron, Poison Hand Training Book 1.* USA. No Publisher listed. Third revised Edition 1963.

Lee, Marion M. (PHD, MPH)., Shen, Jennifer M. (PHD, MPH). *Dietary patterns using Traditional Chinese Medicine principles in epidemiological studies.* San Francisco, CA: *University of California at San Francisco, Department of Epidemiology and Biostatistics, and Department of Family and Community Medicine.* 2008.

Musashi, Miyamoto. *The Book Of Five Rings: Gorin No Sho.* Translation and Commentary by Nikon Services Corporation: Bradford J. Brown, Yuko Kashiwagi, William H. Barrett, and Eisuke Sasagawa. New York, Toronto, London, Sydney, Auckland: Bantam Books. 1982.

Musashi, Miyamoto., Kaufman, Stephen F. *The Book Of Five Rings: The definitive interpretation of Miyamoto Musashi's classic book of strategy.* Tokyo, Rutland, Vermont, Singapore: Tuttle Publishing. 1994.

National Institute of Diabetes and Digestive and Kidney Diseases. "Health Risks of Overweight & Obesity." NIDDK.NIH.gov. February 2018. Accessed September 11, 2021. https://www.niddk.nih.gov/health-information/weight-management/adult-overweight-obesity/health-risks

National Institute of Health. "Parasites associated with pork and pork products." PubMed.gov. August 16, 1997. Accessed September 11,2021. https://pubmed.ncbi.nlm.nih.gov/9501363/

National Institute of Health. "Risk in Red Meat?" NIH.gov. March 26, 2012. Accessed September 11, 2021. https://www.nih.gov/news-events/nih-research-matters/risk-red-meat

Natural Food Pantry. "No Disease Can Exist In An Alkaline Environment." June 16, 2017. Accessed September 11, 2021. https://naturalfoodpantry.ca/blogs/mind-body/no-disease-can-exist-in-an-alkaline-environment

NCBI, NIH. "Anticancer Properties of Graviola (*Annona muricata*): A Comprehensive Mechanistic Review." US National Library of Medicine. National Institute of Health. NCBI.NLM.NIH.gov. July 30, 2018. Accessed September 11, 2021. https://www.ncbi.nlm.nih.gov/pmc/articles/PMC6091294/

NCBI. "LiverTox: Clinical and Research Information on Drug Induced Liver Injury." " NonSteroidal Anti-inflammatory Drugs NSAID's." NCBI.gov. March 18, 2020. Accessed September 11,2021. https://www.ncbi.nlm.nih.gov/books/NBK548614/

Newman, Tim., Seunggu Han, M.D. *All About the Central Nervous Systems*. MedicalNewsToday.com. 2017.

Newsweek Magazine. *Bruce Lee: 75 Years of the Dragon*. New York City, New York USA: Dev Pragad. 2015.

Ngai, Ping Long., Chen, Rongjin. *Kung Fu Quest: Shaolin*. Documentary. 2016.

Nicholas Wade. "Your Body Is Younger Than You Think." New York Times, nytimes.com. August 2, 2005. Accessed September 11, 2021. https://www.nytimes.com/2005/08/02/science/your-body-is-younger-than-you-think.html

NLM. "Nonsteroidal anti-inflammatory drug – induced liver injury – control study in primary care." PubMed.gov. April 18, 2004. Accessed September 11, 2021. https://pubmed.ncbi.nlm.nih.gov/15066135/

PMC Labs. "Poultry and Livestock Exposure and Cancer Risk among Farmers in the Agricultural Health Study." National Institute of Health. PMC Labs. NCBI.NLM.NIH.gov, March 10, 2012, Accessed September 11, 2021, https://www.ncbi.nlm.nih.gov/pmc/articles/PMC3337970/

PubMed. "Potential Animal Health Hazards of Pork and Pork Products." National Institute of Health. PubMed.NCBI.NLM.NIH.gov, April 16, 1997. Accessed September 11, 2021. https://pubmed.ncbi.nlm.nih.gov/9329109/

PubMed. "The Role of Tamarix gallica Leaves Extract in Liver Injury Induced by Rifampicin Plus Isoniazid in Sprague Dawley Rats." PubMed.gov.

January 2, 2018. Accessed September 11, 2021. https://pubmed.ncbi.nlm.nih.gov/28459346/

PubMed. "The Sweet Dangers of Added Sugars." National Institute of Health. PubMed.NCBI.NLM.NIH.gov, June 20, 2019. Accessed September 11, 2021. https://pubmed.ncbi.nlm.nih.gov/31246081/

PubMed."Associations among binge eating behavior patterns and gastrointestinal symptoms: a population-based study." US National Library of Medicine. National Institute of Health. NCBI.NLM.NIH.gov. January 3, 2009. Accessed September 11, 2021. https://www.ncbi.nlm.nih.gov/pmc/articles/PMC2754813/

Rippetoe, Mark., Kilgore, Lon. *Starting Strength*: 2nd Edition. Wichita Falls, Texas USA: The Aasgaard Company. 2007.

Sandra Cabot. MD, "Liver Doctor." LiverDoctor.org. Accessed September 11, 2021. https://www.liverdoctor.com/about-dr-sandra-cabot/

Schwarzenegger, Arnold. Dobbins, Bill. *The New Encyclopedia of Modern Bodybuilding*. New York City, New York USA: Simon & Schuster. 1985, 1998.

Seton, Julia MD. *Psychology Of The Solar Plexus And The Subconscious Mind*. New York: Edward J. Clode. 1914.

Shulze, Dr. Richard ND, MH. *Dr. Shulze's 20 Powerful Steps to a Healthier Life*. California USA: Natural Healing Publications. 2010.

Smith, Richard. "Let Food Be Thy Medicine…" US National Library of Medicine. National Institute of Health. NCBI.NLM.NIH.gov. January 24, 2004. Accessed September 11, 2021. https://www.ncbi.nlm.nih.gov/pmc/articles/PMC318470/

Suzuki, Daisetz Teitaro. *Manual Of Zen Buddhism*. New York, USA: Grove Press Inc. 1960.

Trudeau, Kevin. *Natural Cures: They Don't Want You To Know About*. Alliance Pub Group Inc. 2005.

Trudeau, Kevin. *Your Wish Is Your Command*. Audio CD. Publisher: The Global Information Network. 2009.

Tzu, Sun. Kaufman, Stephen F. *The Art Of War: The definitive interpretation of Sun Tzu's classic book of strategy for the martial artist.* Tokyo, Rutland, Vermont, Boston: Tuttle Publishing. 1996.

University of South Alabama. "Drugs and Health Risks." SouthAlabama.edu. Accessed September 11, 2021. https://www.southalabama.edu/departments/counseling/healthrisks.html

USDA. "Food and Nutrition, Dietary Health." US Department of Agriculture. USDA.gov. Accessed September 11, 2021. https://www.usda.gov/topics/food-and-nutrition/dietary-health

Warburg, Otto Heinrich MD. "Otto Heinrich Warburg." Wikepedia.com. Accessed September 11, 2021. https://en.wikipedia.org/wiki/Otto_Heinrich_Warburg

Wattles, Wallace, D. *The Science Of Getting Rich: How To Make Money and Get The Life You Want.* USA: FAB Publishing. 2018.

Wattles, Wallace, D. *How To What You Want.* USA: Originally Published in 1907. JonRose Publishing. 2016.

WCRF. "Cancer Prevention Recommendations." World Cancer Research Fund. WCRF.org. 2018. Accessed September 11, 2021. https://www.wcrf.org/diet-and-cancer/cancer-prevention-recommendations

WCRF. "Limit Fast Foods." World Cancer Research Fund. WCRF.org. 2018. Accessed September 11, 2021. https://www.wcrf.org/dietandcancer/limit-fast-foods/

WCRF. "Limit Red and Processed Meats." World Cancer Research Fund. WCRF.org. 2018. Accessed September 11, 2021. https://www.wcrf.org/dietandcancer/limit-red-and-processed-meat/

West, Helen RD. "7 Science-Based of Milk Thistle." Healthline.com. January 19, 2018. Accessed September 11, 2021. https://www.healthline.com/nutrition/milk-thistle-benefits

Wikipedia. "Acupuncture." Wikipedia.com. Accessed September 11, 2021. https://en.wikipedia.org/wiki/Acupuncture

Wikipedia. "Meridian (Traditional Chinese Medicine)." Wikipedia.com. Accessed September 11, 2021. https://en.wikipedia.org/wiki/Meridian_(Chinese_medicine)

Wikipedia. "Traditional Chinese Medicine." Wikipedia.com. Accessed September 11, 2021. https://en.wikipedia.org/wiki/Traditional_Chinese_medicine

Yang, Jwing-Ming. *The Root Of Chinese Qigong: Secrets Of Health, Longevity, and Enlightenment.* YMAA Publication Center. 1997.

Yau, MK. "Tai Chi exercise and the improvement of health and well-being in older adults." PubMed.Gov. National Institutes Of Health, 2008. Accessed September 11, 2021. https://pubmed.ncbi.nlm.nih.gov/18487895/

www.ingramcontent.com/pod-product-compliance
Lightning Source LLC
LaVergne TN
LVHW011812060526
838200LV00053B/3748